ASSESSING COMPETENCE
TO CONSENT
TO TREATMENT

Assessing Competence to Consent to Treatment

A Guide for Physicians and Other Health Professionals

THOMAS GRISSO   PAUL S. APPELBAUM
University of Massachusetts Medical School
Worcester, Massachusetts

New York   Oxford
OXFORD UNIVERSITY PRESS
1998

Oxford University Press

Oxford   New York
Athens   Auckland   Bangkok   Bogota
Bombay   Buenos Aires   Calcutta   Cape Town
Dar es Salaam   Delhi   Florence   Hong Kong   Istanbul
Karachi   Kuala Lumpur   Madras   Madrid
Melbourne   Mexico City   Nairobi   Paris
Singapore   Taipei   Tokyo   Toronto   Warsaw

and associated companies in
Berlin   Ibadan

Copyright © 1998 by Oxford University Press

Published by Oxford University Press, Inc.
198 Madison Avenue, New York, New York 10016

Oxford is a registered trademark of Oxford University Press

Library of Congress Cataloging-in-Publication Data
Grisso, Thomas.
Assessing competence to consent to treatment :
aguide for physicians and other health professionals /
Thomas Grisso, Paul S. Appelbaum.
p.   cm.
Includes bibliographical references and index.
ISBN 0-19-510372-6
1. Patient participation.   2. Therapeutics — Decision making.
3. Informed consent (Medical law)   4. Intelligence tests.
I. Appelbaum, Paul S.
II. Title.
[DNLM: 1. Patient Acceptance of Health Care.
2. Mental Competency.
3. Patient Participation.   4. Informed Consent.
5. Decision Making.
W 85 G869a   1998]   R727.42.G75   1998   610.69'6 — dc21
DNLM/DLC   for Library of Congress   97-26915

9 8 7 6 5 4 3 2 1

Printed in the United States of America
on acid-free paper

PREFACE

The assessment of patients' capacities to consent to treatment is one of the most challenging tasks facing clinicians today. This book is designed to help them make that assessment.

Decision-making capacities and their evaluation are of great concern because competent patients — those with adequate capacities — have the right to make profound choices about their medical care. Will a life-sustaining respirator be turned off? Should a decision to pursue a high risk course of treatment be accepted? Can a mildly demented patient designate someone else to make decisions for her as she deteriorates? Competent patients, in keeping with the doctrine of informed consent, will be able to make all these choices about their treatment. In contrast, our society protects incompetent patients from the potential harm of the decisions they might make, appointing others to make the decision for them.

Thus, clinicians in general medical, specialty, and mental health settings are confronted with the need to distinguish between competent and incompetent patients. Despite the dimensions of the issues at stake — literally of life-and-death proportions — they have had relatively little help with this task. The law offers a confusing array of standards that do not apply easily to the situations that clinicians see before them every day. Intricate ethical analyses can be enlightening with regard to the principles underlying the issue of competence, but they

offer little assistance with the practical task of distinguishing competent from incompetent patients. Literature to guide the clinician in
this task is sparse, and much of it is based on authors' idiosyncratic
approaches, of uncertain general validity.

This book is aimed at providing relief to clinicians bewildered by
the task they have been asked to perform. We ourselves are clinicians,
each with almost two decades of experience evaluating decision-
making capacities in clinical settings and performing research to clarify the relation of these capacities to legal questions of competence.
We have tried to bring together here the information that we have
found most useful when we teach colleagues and trainees about the
assessment of patients' decision-making capacities.

In the chapters that follow, we concisely describe the role that competence plays in the doctrine of informed consent, as well as the dimensions of the concept. Based on our review of the law and its ethical foundations, we identify the key abilities related to competence
that lie at the core of any assessment. Then we consider the circumstances in which questions about patients' competence may arise, and
describe in detail how assessments can be conducted. The difficult
process of making judgments about patients' competence is explored.
We conclude with a discussion of how decisions should be made for
patients who lack the competence to choose for themselves.

Throughout this book, our emphasis is on providing information of
practical utility to clinicians. Case examples drawn from our own experience (modified only to preclude identification of patients) are
used liberally to illustrate the application of the principles discussed.
We have limited citations to those references most likely to be of use to
clinicians in thinking about assessment of decision-making capacities.

While formulating our approach to these concepts and tasks, we
have attended to the demands of law, professional ethics, and clinical
practice when assessing patients' decision-making capacities. We cau-
tion readers to recognize that our discussions of relevant law focus
primarily on general legal concepts and, where possible, legal requirements that are found with some regularity across U.S. jurisdictions.
There may be important differences in legal requirements within any
particular jurisdiction, however, and clinicians should seek assis-

tance from local sources of information about law pertaining to competence.

Various sources have contributed to our work in this area. We have been fortunate to have had our research on competence to consent to treatment supported for the last eight years by the Research Network on Mental Health and the Law of the John D. and Catherine T. MacArthur Foundation. The MacArthur Competence Assessment Tool–Treatment (MacCAT-T) described in Chapter 6 and included in the Appendix is one of the products of that work. We are thankful not only for the foundation's continued funding and confidence in our work, but also for the collaborative efforts of our fellow members of the Research Network: Shirley Abrahamson, Richard Bonnie, Pamela Hyde, John Monahan (chair), Stephen Morse, Ed Mulvey, Loren Roth, Paul Slovic, Henry Steadman, and David Wexler. They provided much guidance and sound advice as our conceptual and empirical work in this area unfolded; we are profoundly grateful for their assistance. We are especially indebted to Richard Bonnie, Steven K. Hoge, and John Monahan for reviewing an earlier draft and providing their insights for its improvement. For their fine assistance in preparing the book manuscript, we thank Denise Barrett and Carole Puleo.

Other resources for both of the authors deserve acknowledgment. During this project, Dr. Grisso received support from the Center for Psychosocial and Forensic Services Research at the University of Massachusetts Medical School. He received support from the National Institute of Mental Health (grant RO1-MH37231) for earlier work leading to the present project. While this book was being written, Dr. Appelbaum was the Fritz Redlich Fellow at the Center for Advanced Study in the Behavioral Sciences at Stanford, CA; he acknowledges support from that Center's Foundations Fund for Research in Psychiatry, and from National Science Foundation grant SBR-9022192.

We hope that the trainees and clinicians who use this book will benefit from the clinical and research experiences that we have been privileged to have.

Worcester, Mass.   T. G.
June 1997   P. S. A.

CONTENTS

1

WHY COMPETENCE IS IMPORTANT: THE DOCTRINE OF INFORMED CONSENT

Competence is a pivotal concept in decision making about medical treatment. Competent patients' decisions about accepting or rejecting proposed treatment are respected. Incompetent patients' choices, on the other hand, are put to one side, and alternative mechanisms for deciding about their care are sought. Thus, enjoyment of one of the most fundamental rights of a free society — the right to determine what shall be done to one's body — turns on the possession of those characteristics that we view as constituting decision-making competence.

How competence has come to occupy such a central role in the allocation of rights to persons in the health care system is the focus of this chapter. To understand this situation, we must consider the evolution and current status of the doctrine of informed consent, and the ways in which it reflects deeply held notions about promotion of individual well-being and respect for individual autonomy. In subsequent chapters, our focus shifts to how these abstract principles are integrated into clinical practice.

We begin, however, by considering the way in which these issues present in the clinical setting.

THE CASE OF THE BEWILDERED JANITOR

Frank Scott (a fictitious name), a 37-year-old janitor, was admitted to the neurosurgical unit of a university hospital after being found lying unconscious in a pool of blood on a downtown sidewalk. Witnesses had seen him flashing a roll of $100 bills at a party in a nearby building. When Mr. Scott left the party, he was chased down the street by several men, caught, and beaten about the head. Friends said he had recently sold his car for $800 in cash. His pockets were empty when he was found.

Emergency evaluation at the hospital revealed facial bruises and a basilar skull fracture. Computerized tomography of the head revealed a left frontal epidural hematoma (a blood clot pressing on the brain), with some shift in the midline structures of the brain. When the patient regained consciousness, there was no evidence of focal neurological signs, although he was ataxic when he tried to walk. The neurosurgeons concluded that his condition was stable, but that unless the hematoma were evacuated, the patient risked sudden deterioration, perhaps even death. They discussed the procedure with Mr. Scott, who initially consented, then demurred. A psychiatric consultation was requested to assess the patient's capacities to make a decision about his treatment.

The psychiatric consultant came to the patient's bedside with the neurosurgeon. Mr. Scott, whose manner was oddly cheerful and casual, remembered having seen the neurosurgeon before, although he believed that the doctor had approached him requesting a loan. He knew that he was in a hospital but could not say how he got there or what his medical problem was. The neurosurgeon once more explained in simple terms the patient's condition and the need for surgery, along with the potential risks of the procedure, such as infection. It was clear that the patient had problems attending to the discussion for more than 10 seconds at a time. When questioned about what he had been told, the patient said he had "nerves sticking out of his head," and that the doctors wanted to operate. He did not seem to grasp that he had a blood clot in his head or the exact nature of the surgery.

In further discussion it became apparent that the patient understood that the doctors believed something unfortunate might happen to him if he failed to have the surgery but not what the consequences might be or why. Rather than indicating whether he wanted the surgery or not, the patient said that he thought this was a "heavy decision" that he wanted some time to think over. The impression he gave was not of a thoughtful man, struggling with the risks and benefits of surgery, but of someone who wanted to be rid of people who insisted on talking with him about matters of little consequence.

Ultimately, the consulting psychiatrist concluded that Mr. Scott probably would not be considered competent to make decisions about his treatment. His parents were consulted, and they agreed to consent to the surgery on his behalf. The procedure was performed without complications. When the patient was seen 5 days after surgery, he was able to recount some of the events leading up to his hospitalization, but he had no recollection of the discussions regarding the operation. He was pleased with the treatment he had received, indicating that he thought it had been the right thing to do. The sense remained that he never quite appreciated the seriousness of the condition in which he had been.

CONSENT TO MEDICAL TREATMENT: HISTORICAL EVOLUTION

Let us step back for a moment from Mr. Scott's story to see in a fresh light those elements of the clinical setting that we may have come to take for granted. We are struck by the importance that his caregivers placed on obtaining his agreement to proceed with surgery. There was, after all, no dispute among the physicians with regard to what was indicated from a medical perspective. Failing to evacuate the clot pressing on his brain presented serious risks, including the risk of death. The procedure itself was relatively straightforward, with a very low rate of complications. An objective observer, asked to weigh the risks and benefits of the procedure, would almost certainly agree to go to surgery. Indeed, one could imagine a society in which physicians presented with such a situation simply did what they thought was best for the patient — no questions asked. That society, however, is not ours. It is worth reflecting on the origins of the practices we see illustrated in Mr. Scott's story.

The Era of Simple Consent

Western traditions of respect for individual choice, as exemplified in the long thread of Anglo-American law, have protected the right of persons to decide for themselves whether to undergo medical treatment (Faden & Beauchamp, 1986). This has generally been true regardless of the consequences for the patient that refusal of treatment might entail. The historical record begins in 1767 with the first published English case on consent to treatment, *Slater v. Baker and Stapleton*. The court reported in its decision:

> . . . it appears from the evidence of the surgeons that it was improper to [undertake a procedure involving refracturing a bone that was healing poorly] without consent; this is the usage and law of surgeons . . .

Evidence from legal cases in the United States through the nineteenth century and into the twentieth, as well as case reports that describe doctor–patient interactions, suggest the validity of this conclusion: physicians generally did not undertake treatment without their patients' consent.

This practice of the medical profession appears to have been premised on both philosophical and legal principles. Respect for individual choice was a cornerstone of Enlightenment philosophy, the foundation of modern representative government. John Locke, for example, declared that it was only the free choice of persons to aggregate into a common governing system that conferred on government its legitimacy. Later thinkers, such as John Stuart Mill, denied both to government and to individuals the right to infringe the liberty of citizens without their consent, even for the citizens' own benefit, unless others' rights were at stake. This deeply held sense that freedom from unwanted intrusions on one's liberty — and especially on one's body — is a fundamental element of a civilized society was reflected in the common law of battery. A nonconsensual touching, offensive to the person touched, was actionable at common law, even if the touching were performed with the intent of helping the unconsenting victim. Physicians could be, and were, sued for battery when they undertook treatment over patients' objections.

Although the medical profession was governed by the proscription against unconsented touchings, the requirement for patients' consent before the mid-twentieth century had what we might now consider a decidedly formalistic quality. True, patients who refused treatment were not ordinarily treated against their will. Explicit consent, however, might not always be required. The failure to object to a course of treatment as it was being implemented might be taken as "implied" consent on the part of the patient. Thus, had Frank Scott, who thought his surgeon wanted to borrow money from him, failed to protest as he was being wheeled to the operating room, nineteenth-century standards might have accepted that as adequate evidence of consent.

Moreover, there were no requirements about what patients had to be told before their consent was solicited. Surgeons might name the operative procedure they desired to perform — perhaps in Latin — with no elaboration on what was involved. What would Frank Scott, after all, have made of the information that his doctors recommended a "left frontal craniotomy, with evacuation of an epidural hematoma"? Nor was there any need to discuss the risks of treatment with patients. Indeed, nineteenth-century codes of medical ethics encouraged physicians to withhold information from patients when it might demoralize them or lead them to reject needed care. So, although patients' objections to treatment might have been heeded, their consent was often inferred from their passivity or evoked by incomplete or frankly misleading descriptions of their conditions and the proposed treatment. In contrast to what was to come later, these legal rules of limited scope have been called the doctrine of "simple consent."

The Move to Informed Consent

By the mid-twentieth century, traditional approaches to consent to treatment were coming under greater scrutiny. The severest critics of prevailing practices were the courts. As medicine was becoming more complex, with patients facing an increasing number of options for treatment, the courts grew skeptical about the degree to which simple consent protected patients' underlying interests. How could patients truly control what happened to their bodies when they lacked the simplest information regarding their condition and the options for treatment?

In a series of cases from 1955 to 1972, the courts rejected simple consent in favor of a radically different approach that came to be called "informed consent" (Appelbaum, Lidz, & Meisel, 1987). The new doctrine was premised on the belief that patients had the right to receive sufficient information to make meaningful choices among the options they faced. This represented a shift away from an emphasis on patients' right to be free of unwanted intrusions, which undergirded simple consent. Instead, the courts focused on patients' right to make autonomous decisions, suggesting the importance of being able to select desired options, as well as to reject disfavored ones.

As it evolved, informed consent came to require three elements in treatment decision making: *disclosure of information* by clinicians, within a context that allows *voluntary choice*, made by a patient who is *competent to decide*. In the absence of any one of these elements (which will be considered in more detail shortly), consent is not valid, either ethically or legally. Clinicians who fail to obtain a valid informed consent prior to treatment are liable at law for harms that occur to patients that otherwise would have been avoided. There are a small number of exceptions to this rule. In emergencies, when the time required to inform patients and obtain consent is not available without threatening patients' lives and well-being, these requirements are abrogated. Patients may also waive their rights to disclosure and consent. And in some circumstances in which disclosure itself may be harmful to patients, physicians may have the power to withhold certain information (a power that is called "therapeutic privilege"). Because none of these exceptions applied to Frank Scott's case, his neurosurgeon took considerable trouble to explain to him a good deal about his condition and the proposed operation before soliciting his consent. When it appeared that the patient might not be competent to decide about treatment, substitute consent was pursued from the patient's parents. To understand precisely what occurred between Mr. Scott and his physicians, however, we need to know more about the elements of informed consent.

THE ELEMENTS OF INFORMED CONSENT

Disclosure of Information

One of the very first court decisions on informed consent was *Natanson v. Kline*, a 1960 opinion from the Kansas Supreme Court. It outlined the information that physicians would henceforth be required to convey to patients prior to obtaining their consent. This list is essentially unchanged today. Patients must be told about the *nature and purpose of the proposed treatment* or procedure, its *potential benefits and risks*, and the *alternative approaches* available, along with *their benefits and risks.*

From the beginning, it was evident that merely enumerating the categories of information to be disclosed would not help physicians determine how much of each type of information had to be revealed. How detailed must the description of the proposed treatment be? How many benefits and risks should be discussed with patients? Which alternatives should be revealed, and in what degree of detail? Although none of these questions can be answered with mathematical precision, the courts (and later, legislatures drafting statutes on informed consent) have developed two contrasting approaches to these issues.

The *Natanson* court indicated that physicians were responsible for disclosing that amount of information that a reasonable member of their profession would discuss with patients in a similar situation. This so-called professional standard of disclosure looked to the medical profession, as the group best acquainted with the information available, to determine which information and how much of it should be disclosed to patients. One obvious advantage of the professional standard is that it should be fairly easy for physicians to determine how to fulfill their responsibilities: they need only ascertain the practices of their reasonable colleagues and do the same themselves.

Not everyone was happy with a professional standard of disclosure, however. One of the motivating forces behind the development of informed consent law was the belief that physicians were not sharing enough information with patients to allow them to make meaningful choices. To rely on the medical profession to set the standard of disclosure, therefore, seemed contradictory to the underlying impulse of the doctrine. Thus, as time went on, more and more courts embraced an alternative, patient-oriented standard of disclosure: physicians must disclose the information that a reasonable patient would find material to a decision about the proposed treatment. Although many physicians complained that this "materiality standard" left them in the dark as to what needed to be disclosed, it is now the rule in the majority of states.

Notice that the requirement formulated by the courts focused on physicians' disclosure of information, not patients' understanding of the information. Several courts, early in the development of informed consent, expressed the concern that requiring patients to understand the information disclosed might make physicians leery of treating patients with less-than-perfect comprehension. Nonetheless, it is clear at this point that disclosure must take place in a manner that is designed to facilitate understanding, rather than impede it. In general, this means that medical jargon should be translated into terms that laypeople are likely to grasp, and presented in a format that is conducive to comprehension.

Voluntariness

Because the purpose of informed consent is to help patients to make decisions about their medical care, the use of coercion by medical professionals is obviously antithetical to those goals. What constitutes unacceptable coercion — such that a patient's consent is invalid — has been subject to a good deal less scrutiny than the other two elements of informed consent. It is important to consider both what is and what is not unfairly coercive of patients.

Overt threats by caregivers to retaliate against patients who fail to agree to the proposed course of treatment are clearly coercive and thus invalidate consent. Older physicians tell stories of patients' clothing being taken away from them on hospital wards when they refused to cooperate with treatment; patients were told they could have their clothes back when they went along with doctors' recommendations. That sort of behavior, from the pre-informed-consent days, is unacceptable. Nor can physicians legitimately threaten to withdraw from a patient's care merely because the patient disagrees with the proposed course of treatment. (There may, of course, be circumstances in which treatment is rendered futile by patients' refusal to cooperate; withdrawal in such circumstances may be permissible if undertaken properly.)

Sometimes caregivers withhold their recommendations for treatment from patients for fear that favoring one option over another will be perceived as unfair pressure. Such concern is unwarranted. Indeed, one of the services for which patients come to physicians is some indication of the course of treatment physicians would recommend. Even encouraging patients to pursue a particular option is not coercive, unless unfair threats are involved. Clinicians need not simply lay out the alternatives for patients. They can distinguish among the options they consider more or less viable.

Apparent threats to the voluntariness of patients' decision making can also come from other people in patients' lives. A spouse, for example, may threaten to leave a patient unless he or she agrees to surgery or accepts Antabuse for alcoholism. Such threats are different, however, for the purpose of assessing the validity of a consent, when they come from outside the treatment team. Family members and others in patients' lives are entitled to make demands on them as conditions for continuing relationships. These pressures are simply part of the background that patients bring to the treatment setting. Clinicians need not refrain from initiating treatment because a patient has consented out of concern for the reaction of a loved one.

Competence

Provision of relevant information and absence of coercion are necessary, but not sufficient, conditions for patients to make meaningful choices about treatment. Persons who are unable to utilize the disclosed information because they lack certain basic cognitive capacities are not capable of participating in the process envisioned by the progenitors of informed consent law. At some point, when their impairments become sufficiently severe, we say they are incompetent to make decisions, and they are deprived of that power.

In law, incompetence may be identified in two broad ways. Some persons as a class are considered incompetent as a matter of law (*de jure* or *per se* incompetence). For example, the law considers children incompetent for many types of decisions, partly because of presumptions about their immature cognitive abilities and capacities for judgment. In addition, there are situations in which persons about whom there is a question of their decision-making capacity have already been declared legally incompetent by a court to make similar decisions. In virtually all other cases, however, the question of individuals' competence requires an inquiry into their actual capacities, incompetence being determined on the basis of a demonstrated lack of the requisite functional abilities for the specific individual in question (*de facto* incompetence).

The requirement of competence as a precondition for the exercise of decision-making powers is not peculiar to health law. In general, our society will deny persons the right to make their own decisions if their capacities are sufficiently impaired. Thus, persons can lose the powers to make contracts, give gifts, write a will, decide where to live, and even marry or vote if they are shown to lack the relevant decision-making abilities. Although many of these lines of law have developed independently, and terminologies differ, the criteria applied to determine competence for these tasks are similar at core to those used in the treatment decision-making context.

Chapters 2 and 3 consider which capacities are so critical to good decision making that, in their absence, persons cannot make a meaningful choice, and thus come to be called incompetent. In the remainder of this book, we address issues related to assessing these capacities and how to respond when patients are thought to be incompetent.

Most authors distinguish between *assessments of decision-making capacity*, which health care professionals can conduct, and *determinations of competence*, which are legal judgments left to the courts. Although technically correct, this distinction tends to break down in practice (see Chapter 7). When clinicians determine that a patient lacks decision-making capacity, the practical consequences may be the same as those attending a legal determination of incompetence. For Frank Scott, for example, it meant that his parents were asked to make the decision for or against surgery on his behalf. Thus, in this book, we talk of "decision-making capacities" when we refer to the abilities related to decisions. We use the term "competence," however, to denote the state in which patients' decision-making capacities are sufficiently intact for their decisions to be honored (and conversely for incompetence), regardless of who makes that determination.

THE IMPORTANCE OF COMPETENCE

In describing the requirement that patients be competent to make treatment decisions for their consent to be valid, we noted that this was to ensure that decisions about medical care be made on the basis of "meaningful" choices. This description requires some elaboration. What are the values we are trying to protect — embedded in the concept of a "meaningful choice" — by refusing to accept the decisions of incompetent patients? Two core interests are at stake here (Buchanan & Brock, 1989).

First, as a society, we have an interest in promoting the welfare of our fellow citizens and, concomitantly, in protecting them from harm. Most democratic societies embrace the idea — as a general rule — that each person is best able to determine which choices maximally advance his or her own welfare. This belief is reinforced by the sad experience of those societies that routinely have substituted governmental or other institutional choices for the decisions of individual citizens. Our benevolent concerns, therefore, ordinarily lead us to take a "hands off" approach to the choices people make.

At times, however, the assumption that individual choice is the most likely mechanism to maximize welfare is called into question. When persons are unable to identify their preferences or to select that course of action most consistent with their preferences, the usual relationship between persons' choices and their overall well-being breaks down. Under these circumstances, their decisions, far from being meaningful, may become essentially random. Not only is the general justification for respecting individual choice inapplicable in such cases, but our very concern for their welfare may lead us to do what we ordinarily eschew: deprive them of decision-making power and find alternative means of making choices on their behalf.

Our willingness to take this step, however, is constrained by the second value that underlies the concept of competence: persons' interest in autonomy or self-determination. Western societies embrace autonomy as an ideal not just because the exercise of self-determination is likely to advance personal well-being, but also as a good in itself. Put differently, we might say that persons have an interest in making autonomous decisions *per se*, regardless of whether another decision maker might choose more wisely. Parents who have attempted to select their children's occupations, places of residence, or mates, arguing that their greater experience in life will lead them to avoid the errors to which their offspring are liable, often discover to their chagrin just how firmly held this value is.

What constitutes the exercise of autonomy is a complex philosophical problem that we cannot address in detail here. Not all decisions, however, are autonomous ones. The delirious patient in an intensive care unit who pulls out an intravenous line has not made an autonomous decision. Although the line is uncomfortable and pulling it out will relieve the pain, the patient's behavior is more reflexive than rational. It lacks several of the indicia of autonomous choice, including the abilities to comprehend the current circumstances, to reason about the available options, and to select a course of action. Choices made in the absence of these abilities, or when they are substantially impaired, cannot be said to be autonomous; they are, in the language we used earlier, not meaningful decisions.

Persons who can choose autonomously, however, enjoy the strong presumption that their decisions should be respected. Therefore, the fact that persons have made decisions that are likely to lead to harm — for example, declining antibiotic treatment of endocarditis or electing to have a potentially curable cancer treated with herbal therapy — is an insufficient basis for refusing to accept their choices. Were that not the case, the ideal of self-determination would lie crumpled in the corridors of hospital wards and in outpatient consulting rooms. Rather, the justification for imposing choices on other people is dependent on the impairment of their power of autonomous choice. As the degree of impairment grows, reducing the possibility of self-determination in their cases, we become increasingly justified in substituting other decision-making mechanisms for their choices.

The two values underlying competence — promotion of well-being and autonomy — exist in tension with one another. When people make choices that may lead to harm, we are asked to balance the desire to protect their interests with the value of respecting their self-determination. In general, as the risk of harm increases, the degree of impairment in autonomous decision making required to negate persons' choices decreases. Indeed, there are circumstances in which the risk of harm is so substantial that our society believes it is justified in interfering even with the choices of fully competent persons. The substantial risk of harm from injuries in auto accidents, for example, has led some states to override individual decisions and mandate seat belt use for all occupants of automobiles.

In general, however, and certainly in the case of medical treatment, persons have the right to make decisions that may lead to harm unless their ability to make autonomous choices is so limited that we consider them incompetent. Self-determination, when not substantially impaired, trumps the interest in promotion of well-being and protection from harm. Thus, persons are presumed to be competent to make their own decisions, and the burden of proving otherwise rests on those who would overturn patients' decisions. In this manner, the rules related to decision-making competence protect some of the most important values in our society.

SUMMARY

Informed consent to medical treatment developed out of the concern of the courts that patients have adequate information with which to make meaningful treatment decisions. Information alone, however, is an inadequate predicate to meaningful choice. Patients must also be so situated as to be free of coercion and they must have the capacities to use the information in a rational process of choice. It is from the latter conclusion that the legal and ethical analyses of competence emanate.

Rules governing the assessment of competence reflect a balance between desires to protect persons from potentially harmful decisions, and deeply held beliefs about the inviolability of individual choice. There is no doubt that, in our society, the balance between these two interests is weighted to favor autonomy in decision making, as evidenced by the general presumption of competence in the absence of convincing evidence to the contrary.

Issues related to competence, as we will see in Chapter 2, inevitably arise with regard to a particular decision at a given point in time (Cutter & Shelp, 1991). Focusing on competence-related questions, as we do in this book, risks blurring the reality that informed consent is best seen not as an event that occurs at a single point in time but as a process that pervades the doctor–patient relationship. Except when a discrete treatment of a time-limited condition is at issue (e.g., appendectomy for acute appendicitis), the disclosure envisioned by the law need not, and should not, be transmitted as a whole to patients at the inception of a treatment relationship. Rather, as patients' conditions evolve, new information becomes available, and decisions need to be made, caregivers can disclose the relevant data to patients, solicit and answer their questions, anticipate their concerns, and help apply their preferences to the decision-making process. Moreover, providing information over time may allow patients to assimilate the information more comfortably and completely, thereby maximizing their actual understanding.

It is true, however, that concerns about patients' competence are most likely to arise at particular points along the way, especially when new information is revealed and a decision must be made. The focus in subsequent chapters on these decisional nodes in the consent process should not be taken as implying that these are the only times when informed consent is relevant to the treatment relationship. Indeed, every interaction between patients and caregivers can be used to advance the goal of informed consent: meaningful participation by patients in decisions about their care.

2

THINKING ABOUT COMPETENCE

Clinical assessment of competence to consent to treatment cannot be done by following a set of "cookbook" procedures. It requires an understanding of the concepts underlying competence. Assessing a patient's competence by rote procedures is as problematic as attempting to reach clinical diagnoses with a checklist of criteria but without a theoretical grasp of the constructs on which they are based.

What are the concepts that underlie competence to consent to treatment? What presumptions are reflected in our notions of competence? How do we define its essential features and its foundational characteristics? The first part of this chapter addresses these questions. Then, based on this description of the concepts involved, we outline broad objectives for the assessment of competence to consent to treatment.

Our description of competence is guided substantially by the way in which the law construes it. In clinical practice, it is important that judgments about patients' competence be shaped by legal considerations, as these reflect the rules our society has adopted to protect patients' interests and rights. Fortunately, what we describe here from a legal perspective is consistent with what would flow from an ethical analysis of competence as well.

FIVE MAXIMS OF LEGAL COMPETENCE

Clinicians' thinking about patients' competence should be guided by certain fundamental principles, which we offer here as five "maxims." These principles are not specific to competence to consent to treatment; they can be applied to other types of legal competence as well (e.g., other questions in civil law such as competence to conduct one's general affairs, or competence to stand trial in criminal cases). Therefore, these maxims provide a conceptual link among all types of legal competence, offering the consistency of thought in dealing with them.

These maxims are widely accepted by experts on legal competence and ethical practice. Despite this consensus, they are neither obvious nor well known to many clinicians with limited experience in dealing with questions of competence. Indeed, grasping these maxims will help the clinician go a considerable way toward avoiding some of the more common errors and misconceptions about competence that have been manifested in the past.

Legal Incompetence Is Related to, But Not the Same as, Impaired Mental States

Until quite recently, it was common for clinicians to presume that serious mental illness, mental retardation, or cognitive impairment *per se* rendered a patient incompetent to consent to treatment. This presumption frequently was recognized in the legal system as well. Courts often accepted a clinician's diagnosis of mental illness as all that was required to settle the matter.

The most fundamental, important, and uncontroversial maxim we can offer about the modern concept of legal competence is that this presumption is obsolete. Courts across the land have made it consistently clear that the presence of mental illness, mental retardation, or dementia alone does not render a person incompetent. A patient may be psychotic, seriously depressed, or in a moderately advanced stage of dementia, yet still be found competent to make some or all decisions. Most states' mental health codes specify that even involuntary commitment does not negate the presumption that patients are competent to make treatment (and other) decisions during hospitalization. This is consistent with the ethical imperative that patients' autonomy should not be denied merely because they are ill.

There is, of course, a *relation* between impaired mental states and legal incompetence. A legal finding of incompetence to consent is rare in the *absence* of mental illness, mental retardation, dementia, or other conditions (e.g., traumatic brain injury or delirium induced by toxic or febrile states) that may influence mental and emotional functions involved in decision making. When incompetence is found, it is usually among persons with mental or cognitive disorders. In this sense, the presence of mental disorder or cognitive impairment is often considered a threshold question for the competence judgment, opening an inquiry into whether and how the patient's abilities to make treatment decisions may be impaired.

The assertion that mental illness and cognitive disorders are not synonymous with critical impairment of decision-making abilities is supported by research on the cognitive functioning of persons with these disorders. Our own empirical studies of decision-making abilities among persons with mental illness (Appelbaum & Grisso, 1988, 1995; Grisso & Appelbaum, 1995a, b; Grisso, Appelbaum, Mulvey, & Fletcher, 1995), as well as the work of other researchers, provide support for the presumptions described earlier. We found much variability among persons recently hospitalized for mental illnesses in their abilities to understand disclosures about disorders and treatment options and to reason about them to reach treatment decisions. Some variability was related to diagnosis; for example, patients with major depression performed better than patients with schizophrenia. Of special importance, however, most patients hospitalized with mental illnesses performed as well as research subjects who had no history of mental disorders. Even among patients recently hospitalized for schizophrenia, about one-half of them — and for some decision-making abilities as many as three-quarters — performed as well as a non-ill comparison group.

One might say, therefore, that mental illness increases the *risk* of deficits associated with legal incompetence or mental incapacity but does not create a presumption of incompetence. Whether a person is judged incompetent will depend substantially on the *actual effects* of the person's mental disorder, which is the subject of the next maxim.

Legal Incompetence Refers to Functional Deficits

In questions of competence, the law's fundamental concern is with the effects of patients' mental disorders on their actual cognitive functioning. What is the patient actually able or not able to understand? If the patient has delusional beliefs, how do these beliefs produce deficits in treatment decision making? What is the patient's actual ability for reasoning during decision making? These questions of functioning are central to judgments about patients' competence.

What cognitive abilities and characteristics might be relevant when assessing patients' functioning in decision-making situations? Certainly a number could be nominated: orientation, attention, memory, intelligence, abstract thinking and problem-solving, to name only a few.

As we will see in Chapter 3, however, a set of "legal standards" for competence has evolved as the law has addressed questions of competence over the centuries. These legal standards focus on certain functional abilities on which the law relies to structure its thinking about competence, based on information that clinicians and others can provide about patients' functional deficits or strengths in decision making, including (1) *understanding* of information that is disclosed in the informed consent process, (2) *appreciation* of the information for one's own circumstances, (3) *reasoning* with the information, and (4) *expressing a choice.*

In this book, when we speak of "functional abilities" related to competence, we are referring to these ability concepts. Because of their relation to the legal standards by which competence is judged, they are the foundational concepts in a competence assessment. As the next two maxims will show, however, how those standards are applied depends on something more than the presence of mental impairment and evidence of functional deficits alone.

Legal Incompetence Depends on Functional Demands

When the law considers the question of competence, one of its fundamental concerns is with the person's functional abilities to meet the
demands of a particular "task" or situation. Whether people are considered competent or incompetent will depend in part on the demands of the specific task that they face. The task defines what they
must be able to do, and how well they must be able to do it, in order
to be considered legally competent. This occurs in three ways.

Demands of the task domain. Different areas or domains of functioning in our lives make different demands on our abilities, and we do
not necessarily function equally well in all domains. For example,
capacities for understanding and reasoning are required in order to
master the intricacies of the information superhighway, the rewiring of
a portion of one's home electrical system, and the development of a
good relationship with one's child. Yet the ability to do any one of
these things does not necessarily indicate an ability to do the others.

By the same token, when questions of competence arise, they may
involve only a portion of the domains in which a person functions. In
civil law, for example, courts often must decide people's competence
to make a will, manage their financial affairs, or manage the custody
of their children.

Until recent years, the law tended to perceive individuals simply as
incompetent or competent for all such purposes. In contrast, there is
now wide acceptance of the notion of "specific competencies," in
which competencies for various decision-making domains are not necessarily seen as equivalent. For example, an elderly person with mild
to moderate dementia may be judged incompetent for purposes of
financial budgeting so as to meet monthly expenses. Yet the same
person might be judged competent to decide whether to undergo
elective dental surgery, or to choose between a highly intrusive treatment with excellent prospects and a less intrusive treatment with good
prospects.

Of course, one will encounter cases in which patients' functional
disabilities are so severe that they do, in fact, render them incompe-

tent for all or most types of decisions. The possibility of competence for one purpose but not for another is more likely to arise for patients whose deficits are not so extreme or broad reaching. In these cases especially, the person's incapacities for one purpose should not create a presumption about incompetence for other purposes.

Demands of the case-specific decision. Even within a specific domain of legal competence, such as making decisions about treatment, individual clinical circumstances will vary in the task demands that they make on patients. Various disorders, as well as their treatments, benefits, and risks, will be more or less complex and far-reaching in their consequences. This makes different demands on patients' abilities of comprehension, appreciation, and reasoning. For this reason, a patient may be found competent to make decisions about one treatment situation but not another.

A specific type of treatment also may vary in its benefits and risks, depending on differences among patients in their clinical conditions or medical histories. Such differences may make the clinical picture more or less difficult for patients to comprehend or to weigh, even when they all face the same treatment. It follows that clinicians must consider the nature of decision-making problems that patients face, in light of patients' own disorders and relevant treatment options, to grasp the demands made on their patients' abilities.

Situational variations in demands. Patients' decisions about potential treatments do not occur in a vacuum. In addition to the nature of the treatment choices they face, the medical and social contexts in which they must decide will increase or decrease the demands of their decisional tasks.

For example, some treatment decisions must be made quickly because the patient's illness or trauma requires immediate intervention to avoid rapid and fatal deterioration. In other cases, clinicians can employ low-risk analgesic or stabilizing interventions that allow a safe delay of more definitive procedures for several days, giving patients time to consider the options. In general, the latter situation places less demand on patients' decision-making abilities.

Social circumstances may influence task demand. Some patients must decide about their treatment alone; others may be assisted by family members or friends who can share with them the burden of thinking through the options.

Therefore, the situational and interpersonal contexts in which patients' treatment decisions are made can be important determinants of the demands placed on their decision-making abilities. Some of these determinants arise naturally from the circumstances of their disorder, whereas others can be manipulated to increase or reduce the demands that patients face.

Summary of the task demand maxim. Overall, the task demand maxim has important implications when it is considered alongside the maxim on functional deficits. Placed together, they suggest that competence is not simply dependent on a person's abilities, but on the *match or mismatch between the patient's abilities and the decision-making demands of the situation that the patient faces.* This contrasts sharply with the more traditional view, now outdated, that competence simply reflects the patient's clinical or psychological condition.

This conclusion has numerous important implications. First, it means that there is no absolute level of ability that defines competence or incompetence. The degree of ability that is necessary in order to be considered competent will depend in part on how much is demanded. This will vary from case to case; no single "criterion" will apply across all cases. Two patients may have equal degrees of decision-making ability, yet one may be considered competent and the other incompetent, if the decisions that they face are very different in their demands.

Second, it means that an assessment for legal competence often cannot be based solely on an investigation of the person's functional abilities. In many cases it will also require inquiry into the decision-making demands of the situation.

Third, it means that there are two ways to think about responding to a patient's potential incompetence. One may try to increase the person's functional abilities (e.g., reduce the use of medications that may be contributing to a delirium). Alternatively, consistent with our discussion of "situational variation," one may try to decrease the decision-making demands of the situation. We will review the use of this strategy in detail in Chapter 5, when we discuss ways to assist patients who have limited abilities so as to avoid restricting their decision-making autonomy whenever possible.

Indeed, we will return to this "person-task" concept of legal competence many times in this book, as we describe the choice of assessment methods, data collection, interpretation of data, and conclusive judgments about competence.

Legal Incompetence Depends on Consequences

Law and ethical practice require that we interfere as little as possible with persons' right to make autonomous decisions about their lives. Some limits on this right, however, are justified legally and ethically when individuals with mental conditions that impair their decision making are likely to suffer harm if their choices are honored. A consideration of the consequences of abiding by the decisions of patients with mental impairment, therefore, properly plays a role in judgments about competence (and acceptance of patients' choices) or incompetence (and assignment of choice to someone who will decide on patients' behalf).

This is done by adjusting upward or downward the degree of disability that is required in order to categorize patients as incompetent, depending on the degree of harm associated with their probable choice. This "degree" of ability is often called the *threshold* for competence; for example, a demand for greater ability sets a "higher threshold" that must be met to conclude that the person is competent to decide. A better grasp of how and on what bases thresholds for competence vary can be seen by considering several types of treatment situations.

High benefit, low risk treatment. As a general rule, a *lower* threshold for competence is set when a patient is *accepting* a treatment option that is much needed (the patient is suffering or will suffer if not treated), is very likely to be ameliorative (suffering is very likely to be relieved), and presents only low to moderate risk of negative effects (the cost of relief of suffering is low). Conversely, a somewhat *higher* threshold for competence may be required for patients who are *refusing* the same type of treatment option. The logic for this difference lies in the value our society places on the best medical interests of the patient, and the desire not to deprive patients of that treatment when their refusals may be the product of impaired thinking.

Judgments about patients' competence to accept or refuse medications to treat pneumonia probably fall into this category. So do many surgical interventions for which risks and anticipated negative consequences are low to moderate, together with a high likelihood of success in averting current or future disability (e.g., treating fractures of the limbs).

Low benefit, high risk treatment. This situation represents the mirror image of the circumstances addressed above: patients are deciding to accept treatments that are unlikely to yield significant benefits, and either pose substantial risks of adverse effects, or are likely to leave them at the mercy of their disease processes. Examples might include the choice of herbal enemas as a treatment for colon cancer, or the use of a heroic intervention — like an artificial heart — without a track record of success. Our interest in protecting people from harm might legitimately lead us to demand *higher* thresholds for competence in these cases.

Low to moderate benefit, low to moderate risk treatment. In some cases, patients will be choosing treatments that may yield some benefit to them, and only a moderate degree of risk from adverse outcomes. As a corollary, foregoing such treatment will not induce substantial harm. As a society, we are largely indifferent to patients' choices in such circumstances. Thus we require only a low level of abilities before accepting patients' decisions. This is another way of saying that in almost all circumstances, the choice should be theirs. Much the same might be said for situations in which the treatment that is required to save a person's life will have serious negative consequences even if the treatment is successful (e.g., amputation of a gangrenous leg in a diabetic who has already lost the opposite leg).

In all of the treatment circumstances we have considered here, which by no means exhaust the possibilities, the clinician should think about a requirement for a "higher threshold" for competence in relative terms, and in the context of the mental condition that is impairing a patient's decision-making abilities. A "lower" threshold means that greater impairment is allowed before the patient is considered incompetent, and a "higher" threshold means that less impairment is allowed. But even a high threshold rarely implies abilities beyond those of the average person who is without mental disorder.

When clinicians consider the effects of potential consequences on their judgments about patients' competence, they encounter a number of issues that our description does not answer. For example, clinicians will differ in their interpretations of whether a treatment presents "high benefits" or "high risks." In Chapter 7 we will have ample opportunity to examine in more detail how the consequences of treatment options come into play in specific situations.

Legal Incompetence Can Change

At one time legal incompetence was considered to be a more or less enduring status. Once a patient had been declared incompetent to make a treatment decision, there was little reason ever to revisit the question.

Modern mental health law, however, does not construe incompetence as a static condition. It recognizes that people's cognitive and emotional states may change or fluctuate, influencing changes in critical decision-making abilities. In our studies of mentally ill patients' capacities for treatment decision making, we examined changes in their performance during the first two weeks of their hospital treatment for acute disorders (Grisso, Appelbaum, Mulvey, & Fletcher,

1995). We found that patients with schizophrenia who improved significantly from admission to retest on measures of severity of symptoms (e.g., Brief Psychiatric Rating Scale) also improved in their performance on measures of understanding and reasoning in hypothetical treatment situations. Thus, the law's approach seems to comport with what we know about patients' decision-making abilities.

Changes in patients' capacities may occur for reasons other than response to treatment. In some cases they may vary from day to day, fluctuating in response to changes in their status: for example, increases and decreases in orientation and attention due to fluctuations in febrility.

Because incompetence refers to a current condition and does not necessarily imply an enduring status, it is important that patients considered incompetent at a particular point in time should be reassessed periodically. When the clinical status of incompetent patients improves, ethical and legal considerations impel us to consider whether they have the capacity to resume a role in making decisions about their treatment. Similarly, deteriorating conditions may require reconsideration of the status of patients who formerly were judged competent.

Summary: A Definition of Incompetence

The five maxims can be used to produce a definition of incompetence. The key words of the maxims are italicized:

> Incompetence constitutes a status of the individual that is defined by *functional* deficits (due to *mental illness, mental retardation, or other mental conditions*) judged to be sufficiently great that the person *currently* cannot meet the *demands* of a specific decision-making situation, weighed in light of its potential *consequences*.

This specific definition will not be found in law. Yet it is consistent with both ethical and legal notions of competence as they are described in leading texts and case law.

IMPLICATIONS FOR ASSESSMENT OBJECTIVES

Given the concept of competence as we have described it, one can begin to see what types of information should be obtained and considered in evaluating the competence of patients to consent to treatment. As we noted in Chapter 1, evaluating patients' competence is not necessarily an "event." In good clinical practice, it is an ongoing process that is a part of the day-to-day treatment relationship between doctor and patient. In either sense, an assessment of a patient's decision-making competence requires the following elements.

Assessing Psychopathology

No evaluation for competence can be complete without a thorough *clinical knowledge of the patient's psychopathology.* Special attention is required regarding the presence, severity, and specific effects of psychopathologic symptoms, and awareness of how they might influence mental or emotional processes involved in patients' efforts to make decisions about treatment. We discuss the relation between various psychopathological conditions and decision-making abilities in Chapters 3 and 4.

Observing Functioning in Decision-Making Tasks

One's assessment of competence should, whenever possible, include direct observation of the patient's *functioning in tasks involving decision-making abilities.* In general, we take unnecessary risks if we make judgments about patients' decision-making abilities solely on the basis of our knowledge of their psychopathology. As noted in the first maxim, not all mental conditions — even serious ones — render patients incapable of making meaningful decisions. Moreover, our empirical knowledge of the actual relations between specific symptoms of mental disorder and decision-making abilities is not well developed.

There will be cases, of course, in which such matters are not seriously in doubt: for example, persons who are comatose, have advanced dementias, or suffer from acute psychotic conditions, whose symptoms grossly and obviously impair their functioning for almost any purpose. In cases like these, inference about functional decision-making deficits based on clinical symptoms alone often will be warranted. In cases involving less than extreme clinical conditions, however, one should avoid substituting such inferences for direct observation of patients' decision-making abilities. If we do not, we run the risk of wrongly depriving some patients of their right to make decisions of which they are capable, or failing to protect some patients from the potential harm of their decisions made incompetently.

In Chapter 3, we will see the types of functional decision-making abilities that should be assessed. Methods for their assessment will be described in Chapters 5 and 6.

Recognizing Functional Task Demands

In most cases, the assessment is not concluded with an evaluation of the patient. One must also take stock of the *demands that the situation places on the patient's abilities*. This will require a consideration of the nature and complexity of the illness and its alternative treatments, as well as the range of situational variables that may augment or reduce the difficulty of the decision-making task for the patient. Later we discuss how these considerations can be incorporated into one's assessment of the patient's functional abilities (Chapter 5), how they can be used in making judgments about competence (Chapter 7), and in some cases, how such factors can allow one to create conditions that reduce the need to judge a patient incompetent.

Considering Consequences

Decisions about the threshold to employ in making the judgment about competence or incompetence will require information concerning the *probable consequences of the patient's treatment choice*. Generally this information will be part of clinicians' knowledge within their field of medical specialization. Probable outcomes of treatment options, however, also depend in part on medical, psychological, and social characteristics of the specific patient in question. Obtaining such information will be described in Chapter 5 and 6, and its use in making competence judgments will be explored in Chapter 7.

Employing Reassessment

The potential for change in patients' competent or incompetent status suggests that periodic *reassessment* should be a formal objective of many evaluations for competence to consent to treatment. We will see this in Chapter 8 in the context of substituted decision making for incompetent patients.

SUMMARY

In this chapter we described five maxims of legal competence that are critical for understanding competence as a concept. They emphasized the importance of:

- *Functional abilities* in defining competence;
- *Mental disorders as explanations* for deficits in abilities, but not as sufficient conditions alone to address the question of competence;
- The *demands* that situations place on patients' functioning;
- The *consequences* of patients' decisions for their welfare; and
- Recognition that patients' *capacities may change.*

We then identified several essential features of assessments for patients' competence that parallel these maxims:

- Assessing *functional abilities* related to decision making;
- Assessing *psychopathology*;
- Determining *task demands*;
- Considering *consequences* of patients' decisions; and
- Employing *reassessment* of functioning.

Among these aspects of an assessment for competence, assessing relevant functional abilities related to decision making plays a central role. Identifying the relevant functional abilities is the focus of Chapter 3.

3

ABILITIES RELATED TO COMPETENCE

At the end of Chapter 2, we noted that three kinds of information usually are needed for making judgments about patients' decision-making capacities: (1) the patient's clinical condition, (2) the patient's functioning in tasks involving decision-making abilities, and (3) the specific demands of the patient's treatment situation. Here in Chapter 3 we focus on the second kind of information; we identify and define the types of decision-making abilities that are especially relevant for the competence assessment. Specifically when and how these abilities should be assessed will be discussed in Chapters 4 to 6.

There are four functional abilities that we recommend as the focus of assessments for competence to consent to treatment:

- The ability to *express a choice;*
- The ability to *understand* information relevant to treatment decision making;
- The ability to *appreciate* the significance of that information for one's own situation, especially concerning one's illness and the probable consequences of one's treatment options; and
- The ability to *reason* with relevant information so as to engage in a logical process of weighing treatment options.

Why these specific abilities? Many ways of categorizing, labeling, and defining abilities relevant for treatment decision making have been expressed by courts and legislatures, national panels of policy experts, theorists in the ethics of informed consent, authors providing guidance for clinical evaluations of competence, and — for decision making in general — by psychological theorists and researchers who study cognitive functioning. Definitions have differed from one authority to another. For example, not all courts use exactly the same set of abilities, and ethicists differ about the proper way to conceptualize the critical abilities associated with competence to consent.

Our selection and definitions of these four concepts were developed after a thorough review of the case law and literature on competence. The starting point was Roth, Meisel, and Lidz's (1977) well-known analysis of legal standards for competence to consent to treatment. Our further review of current laws produced refinements in those definitions (Berg, Appelbaum, & Grisso, 1996). In addition, we took into consideration the scholarly analyses of treatment competence by leading medical ethicists (e.g., Buchanan & Brock, 1989; Faden & Beauchamp, 1986), definitions produced by important commissioned studies (e.g., President's Commission, 1982), and clinical views — based on practice and research — relevant to assessment of competence.

Our objective was to develop and define a set of concepts that would cover the critical range and types of abilities that are cited consistently — often under dissimilar nomenclature — by these various authorities. As we describe the abilities, we will point out the ways in which our terms or definitions reflect those that are provided in law or by theorists in medical ethics, as well as any important ways in which they differ.

In beginning to review these ability concepts in detail, it helps to keep in mind that there is no simple relationship between a person's status with regard to these abilities and the judgment that a person is competent to consent to treatment. There are two reasons why this is so.

First, patients' status on these abilities is not an all-or-none matter. Rarely can it be said that a patient does or does not possess one of these abilities; usually patients manifest all of them, but in varying degrees. The question, then, is whether a patient functions sufficiently in these areas of ability to allow a judgment that he or she is competent to decide about treatment. How well the patient must function, of course, will also require a consideration of the nature of the decision to be made (e.g., its complexity and risks), as well as of the clinical condition of the patient. Therefore, the patient's abilities are a very important part of the information with which we work when making judgments about competence, but they are only part of the overall picture; simply knowing the patient's status on the abilities does not by itself decide "competence" or "incompetence."

The second reason that there is no simple relationship between the four abilities and competence is that not all of the ability concepts will be applied in all competence judgments. Some courts, for example, may employ only the ability to understand what is involved in the treatment situation when judging a patient's legal competence. Others may employ all four concepts, requiring a level of adequacy on all of them commensurate with the nature of the treatment decision that the patient faces. Whether one, all, or only some of these abilities are used will depend on the legal or ethical standards that are applied in various jurisdictions. In our view, both empirical evidence and ethical concerns should urge us to attend to all of these abilities in competence evaluations. But one should recognize that, in practice, not all of them uniformly will be "required."

On one point, however, case law and the ethical literature are almost entirely in agreement. As you look at the list of ability concepts outlined earlier, you will notice that they all refer to what goes into treatment decision making, not to what comes out of it. In other words, they refer to how the choice is made, not to the nature of the choice itself. Virtually all legal and ethical perspectives on competence to consent to treatment agree that whether a patient's choice would be considered wise by most people is not a requirement for competence to consent to treatment. Therefore, we do not include anything like an "ability to make the correct or wisest choice."

This absence of a concept defining the "correctness" of choice is not because the quality of the patient's choice is irrelevant to the competence judgment. Often it is the potentially dangerous outcome of what appears to be an inadvisable choice that signals us to raise the question of the patient's competence. Yet a "bad" choice is not a basis for judging the patient incompetent, if the patient's abilities on the dimensions we are describing here are sufficiently intact. This is related to a basic value that was discussed in Chapter 1. Society's interest in protecting the rights of patients to make autonomous choices requires that their decisions be respected unless they are substantially deficient in their abilities to make the choice. To presume their incompetence simply on the basis of the eccentricity or inadvisability of their choice would jeopardize that fundamental freedom.

Let us turn now to examine the ability concepts that are critical for assessing competence to consent to treatment. For each of these abilities, our discussion in this chapter:

- Defines it as a concept consistent with medical ethics and law;
- Interprets its relation to medical and psychological concepts; and
- Identifies its implications for assessments to address questions of competence to consent to treatment.

Throughout our discussion, we often capitalize the first letter of terms referring to these four abilities (e.g., "Understanding"). This makes it clear that as the term is being used at that point, it refers to our specific definition of the ability, not to the more general sense of the term in everyday discourse.

EXPRESSING A CHOICE

A 57-year-old man who recently had emigrated to the United States from central Europe was functioning well until 2 years prior to admission, when he began to develop symptoms of depression. Treatment with medication was unavailing. When a consultant sought him out to discuss possible treatment with electroconvulsive therapy, she found him pacing up and down the hall of the psychiatric unit. As she approached him, he brushed past her, ran into his room, and lay down on the bed, only to get up spontaneously a minute later and, taking unusually large steps, walk to the other end of the hall. This cycle was repeated many times. While lying on the bed, he kept his eyes tightly closed, as if to shut out all those around him. Mostly he was unresponsive to attempts at conversation. Occasionally, though, he would respond to a question, almost at random, telling the consultant his age at one point, and the town he lived in at another. At no point would he respond to any questions about his mental state, understanding of treatment options, or opinions about what course of treatment he might prefer.

Expressing a Choice as a Competence Concept

When patients are unable, as a result of illness, to reach a decision or to indicate to their caregivers what course of treatment they desire, courts and ethicists uniformly have considered them to be incompetent to make treatment decisions. As a legal matter, this requirement is a "threshold" issue; if patients are unable to Express a Choice, usually there is no need to consider their status regarding other abilities. On the other hand, it is rare that persons will be considered competent merely because they can state a preference, given that they have serious deficits in other abilities that we review below. This would set a very low threshold according to which any person who would be considered competent to decide merely on the basis of the ability to signal "yes" or "no," regardless of the quality of thought behind the response.

Although there may be situations involving urgent intervention in which the ability to Express a Choice is sufficient to accept the patient's treatment choice, in ordinary cases the fact that patients have "passed" this requirement does not settle the question of their competence. To "fail" it, however, usually will signify insufficient capacity (and often legal incompetence) to participate meaningfully in the process of deciding about treatment.

Clinical Interpretation of the Concept

Some patients may be unable to state their preferences simply because, at the moment, their disabilities render them incapable of saying or otherwise communicating anything at all. This would be the case, for example, with patients who are comatose or those who are exhibiting catatonic symptoms secondary to psychosis.

Others are able to speak but seem unable to choose — to make up their mind. Thus patients might be considered unable to Express a Choice if, during several consecutive days, they are so ambivalent that they can neither commit to a choice nor elect to assign the decision to someone else. In other cases, patients may vacillate between consent and refusal for medical procedures, thereby producing a clinical stalemate.

> A mildly mentally retarded man was admitted to a general hospital for surgery following damage to his hip in an auto accident. He had a history of hospital admissions for brief periods of psychotic decompensation, but these symptoms were not apparent at admission. His physical condition was stable and he was placed in preoperative traction. He was able to say what he did or did not want. After an explanation of the alternatives, he consented to a hip replacement procedure, and surgery was scheduled for the next morning. During preoperative procedures, however, he suddenly told the nurses that he did not want the surgery. When approached that afternoon, he again consented, then later withdrew his consent once more. This pattern was repeated for 3 days, consent being withdrawn each time the surgery was imminent. The likelihood of satisfactory surgical results diminished each day that the procedure was delayed. After psychiatric consultation, he was deemed incompetent and his parents were asked to make a decision on his behalf.

Implications for Competence Assessment

If the patient cannot express a preference at all, this will usually become obvious in the course of routine attempts to talk to the patient. Cases involving ambivalence or vacillation, however, may not be apparent until the patient needs to make the decision. In these cases, the inability to Express a Choice may only be observed when the information about treatment is explained and an attempt is made to elicit the patient's choice.

The mere fact that a patient cannot speak does not necessarily signify an inability to communicate a decision. Some patients may be able to express a choice in nonverbal ways, for example, in writing or by giving signals with their hands or eyes in response to questions. Exploring these alternatives may be another objective of a competence assessment, as we will see in Chapter 5.

Moreover, some patients with poor English skills may lack the ability to communicate with their caregivers until an interpreter is provided. Indeed, given that the patient in our first case example in this section was an immigrant, his clinician decided to invite his mother and brother to the hospital to see if they could better communicate with him in his native tongue. Only when their efforts were also unavailing did she conclude that the patient's inability to communicate was due to his psychiatric disorder.

UNDERSTANDING

> A 35-year-old acutely psychotic woman, admitted to a psychiatric facility just the day before, was evaluated for treatment with medication. Discussing the options with her, the attending psychiatrist told her that the medication he recommended was likely to help her feel less afraid of others (she had paranoid delusions about people trying to get into her apartment) and that she would be taking the medication orally each morning around breakfast time. She appeared to be listening but said only "yes" whenever asked if she understood the disclosure. Nevertheless, she consented to take the medication. Later in the day, a nurse reported that the patient asked her if the new vitamin pills she would be taking with her breakfast would give her more energy.

Understanding as a Competence Concept

As described in Chapter 1, the doctrine of informed consent includes the notion that patients making decisions about treatment must have available to them the body of relevant information. The disclosure component of the informed consent doctrine requires the health professional to describe the disorder, potential ways to treat it, and their benefits and disadvantages in a way that is likely to maximize the patient's comprehension of them.

Even with the clinician's best efforts, however, some patients are unable to grasp what they are told, thereby failing to acquire the information they need in order to deal meaningfully with the treatment decision. When patients' mental disorders or disabilities seriously impair their ability to comprehend, they may fail to meet the Understanding requirement for competence to consent.

Courts often use this concept in making competence determinations. In fact, among the four ability concepts we review here, Understanding is the most common ability on which legislatures rely and to which judges refer in their competence judgments. It is universally identified as essential in discussions of the ethics of competent consent. Patients are expected to be able to understand that information which must be disclosed under the law of informed consent.

Clinical Interpretation of the Concept

As basic as the concept of Understanding may seem, the psychological processes related to it are not easily defined. A person's accurate assimilation of information involves a complex series of events. First the information must be received as presented, a process that is influenced not only by sensory integrity, but also by perceptual functions such as attention and selective awareness. Whatever is received then undergoes cognitive processing and is encoded in a manner consistent with the person's existing fund of information and concepts, which in turn influences how, and how well, the message is recorded and stored in memory.

Not surprisingly, the concept of Understanding is related in part to a person's general level of intelligence. Persons with limited intelligence or mental retardation may require special consideration when one is describing treatments to them or assessing their competence. Their limitations by themselves do not necessarily render them incompetent according to this standard; persons with mental retardation vary considerably in their capacities to comprehend information, and some treatment situations are easier to comprehend than others. But their limited intellectual capacities place them at greater risk of inadequate comprehension in the informed consent dialogue.

Many studies have documented difficulties in cognitive functions associated with comprehension among persons with acute mental disorders, especially those with schizophrenia (e.g., Clare, McKenna, Mortimer, & Baddeley, 1993; Gold & Harvey, 1993). In our own studies (Grisso & Appelbaum, 1995b), patients recently admitted to psychiatric units with diagnoses of schizophrenia or major depression sometimes manifested very poor comprehension of treatment disclosures compared to persons of similar socioeconomic status but with no illness. The study also showed, however, that one cannot judge patients' capacities to understand simply on the basis of their psychiatric diagnoses. For example, compared to their non-ill counterparts, a *greater proportion* of patients with schizophrenia (about 25%) were impaired in Understanding, but the *majority* did not comprehend less than the comparison group.

Chronic mental disorders and mental disabilities, however, are by no means the only (or even primary) potential causes of deficits in patients' abilities to understand treatment disclosures. A very wide range of medical conditions may place patients at risk of impaired ability to understand relevant information. Consider again the complex sensory, perceptual, and cognitive phenomena involved in the process of achieving understanding of what one is told. Many medical conditions can have a substantial negative influence on these functions. Physical trauma may have both direct (e.g., tissue damage to the structures involved) and indirect (e.g., decrement in overall level of alertness) influences on sensorium and cognitive processes. The ability to comprehend also can be impaired by some medications. In addition, a patient's attempts to adapt psychologically to anxiety concerning a medical condition may temporarily impair the person's ability even to receive and process information about the disorder.

A 69-year-old widow with a history of diabetes was admitted to the hospital for treatment of an ischemic right middle finger.

The problem was apparently due to constriction of the blood vessels caused by overactivity of the sympathetic nervous system. Attempts to block the nerve signals by injecting a local anesthetic into the stellate ganglion were successful on two occasions, but each time when the block wore off, the vasoconstriction returned. Thus, the surgeons proposed to ablate the stellate ganglion, hoping that would result in permanent relief. Although the patient initially consented to the procedure, she subsequently withdrew her consent, and later vacillated back and forth. She appeared terrified by the prospect of surgery. A psychiatric consultant found that the patient seemed lucid and intelligent, but ended the discussion when the consultant began to speak about the possible risks of surgery, saying that she simply did not want to hear about it. Attempts to continue led to her becoming agitated and leaving the room.

Unlike this patient, others overwhelmed by anxiety may display more subtle manifestations, such as selectively failing to attend to information about risks, filtering it in such a way that it seems not to have been received. If such conditions persist in causing patients serious difficulties in grasping the essential messages in a disclosure of treatment information, they may impair Understanding as it relates to patients' competence to consent to treatment.

Implications for Competence Assessment

As the most common requirement applied to questions of patients' competence, Understanding generally will be assessed in all cases in which the patient meets the requirement for Expressing a Choice. The person's general capacity for understanding (i.e., general intelligence) may be clinically relevant for this assessment, but usually it will not be sufficient. Our assessment approach asks the clinician to examine directly the degree to which the patient appears to have understood the information in the disclosure itself. A knowledge of patients' general intellectual capacities often will suggest the likelihood that they are *capable* of comprehending that information, but assessment of what they think the clinician has told them indicates more directly what they *actually* comprehend.

In Chapters 5 and 6, we discuss methods for the direct assessment of what patients understand about treatment disclosures. All such methods, however, have their limitations. Even with direct questioning and observation, we must often infer whether the sensory, perceptual, and cognitive processes involved in acquiring information have resulted in adequate understanding. We determine that people have grasped our meaning when they do or say something that we would expect of persons who have assimilated the information as we meant to convey it.

Sometimes this provides us with an unambiguous basis for concluding that they do or do not understand. But there are instances in which a person's behavior or words may be misleading. This is because another psychological process is involved in producing the evidence. To tell us what they understand, patients must decode their thoughts to form words and phrases that convey what they know. If what they tell us seems to misrepresent the information we gave them, it may simply be due to their difficulties in communicating what they know, not their lack of knowledge. This might require that clinicians develop alternative ways to assess their comprehension that do not rely so heavily on their verbal expressive abilities.

The ability to remember what one has been told is an essential part of Understanding. If information has not been "stored" in a manner that facilitates recall at the time one is making a decision, the relevant information is not available to satisfy the Understanding requirement. For purposes of assessing Understanding as it relates to competence to consent, however, not all types of memory are equally relevant. Some research studies, for example, have found that several days to weeks after treatment disclosures and patients' consent, patients with both medical and mental illnesses often are not able to recall critical information about the treatment options. For purposes of the Understanding standard, however, the important question about memory is whether a person is able to recall relevant information at the time the treatment decision is made. Long-term memory is relevant only when patients are asked to make their decisions several days after disclosure without further discussion with the clinician.

In summary, when and how to assess Understanding presents a number of challenges for clinicians. How to meet those challenges is a primary focus of Chapters 4 to 6.

APPRECIATION

Suffering from the effects of peripheral vascular disease, a 71-year-old woman was admitted to the hospital with gangrene of the three middle toes on her left foot. The residents on the surgical unit explained to her the likelihood that, without amputation of the distal part of her foot, the infection would spread, leading either to subsequent amputation of her leg or, if treatment were still withheld, to her death. She was able to recount everything she was told but refused to proceed with the surgery. When the residents asked why, she explained that, although she thought the doctors were sincere in their desire to help her, they nevertheless were mistaken about the nature of her condition. Her toes were not gangrenous, but simply dirty. If the nurses would wash her toes, which she herself couldn't reach, they would no longer be black and she could go home. Washing her toes and informing her that they were still black did not change her view of the situation; she continued to claim that it was dirt and not gangrene that was the cause of the problem.

Appreciation as a Competence Concept

In dealing with questions of competence, courts and ethicists alike often have examined more than patients' Understanding. They have asked also whether patients (1) acknowledge, or appreciate, that they are suffering from the disorder with which they have been diagnosed, and (2) acknowledge the consequences of the disorder and of potential treatment options for their own situation. We refer to this as the *Appreciation* requirement for competence to consent.

The case of the woman with gangrenous toes provides an example of the conceptual difference between the Understanding and Appreciation requirements. Here the woman appears fully to grasp the meaning of what has been disclosed to her. But she appears not to *believe* that what she has been told applies to her condition. In other words, she understands that death is a likely consequence of failure to amputate gangrenous toes. But she does not accept that her toes are gangrenous, so she does not appreciate the relevance or significance of the information for her situation as she prepares to make her treatment decision.

In cases like this, courts often use an Appreciation requirement that results in a finding of incompetence despite the person's adequate Understanding. The degree to which courts apply this concept, however, is difficult to determine. One encounters cases in which lack of Appreciation would appear to explain a court's decision, yet the court does not expressly state that this was the basis for its finding of incompetence. Similarly, authorities in bioethics and informed consent do not always use the term Appreciation in the way that we are defining it. Sometimes it is used to refer to understanding that goes beyond a factual grasp of consequences to an experiential sense of what the consequences would "really" entail — for example, "what it would be like and 'feel' like to be in possible future states and to undergo potential alternatives" (Buchanan & Brock, 1989, p. 24).

Our meaning of Appreciation is more like that of authorities (e.g., Appelbaum & Roth, 1982; President's Commission, 1982; Roth, Appelbaum, Sallee, Reynold, & Huber, 1982) who use the term in reference to people who, because of cognitive deficits or emotional states, fail to accept the relevance of their disorders or potential treatment consequences for their own circumstances. They hold *"patently false beliefs"* (Saks, 1991), often as a result of denial, distortion, or delusions, that what they are told is not true for them.

Nor do all ethicists conceptualize Understanding and Appreciation as separate abilities related to competence. Several authorities, for example, have preferred to think of people's beliefs, in contrast to their comprehension of what they have been told, as a second kind of understanding or as a second component within a concept called Understanding (e.g., Buchanan & Brock, 1989; Faden & Beauchamp, 1986).

Despite the fact that Understanding and Appreciation are related conceptually, we believe that framing Appreciation as a separate concept has several benefits. First, legal and regulatory definitions related to competence often do so (Berg, Appelbaum, & Grisso, 1996). The President's Commission on Ethical Issues in Medicine and Biomedical and Behavioral Research (1982) referred to capacities to "understand and appreciate," implying that they were sufficiently different to warrant consideration as separate concepts. Similarly, the final report of the British Law Commission (1995) on mental incapacity and the law has cited the value of analyzing decision-making capacity not only in terms of abilities related to "comprehending and retaining information," but also in terms of "believing it" (p. 37). Second, separating Understanding and Appreciation identifies more clearly for clinicians the importance of attending to both abilities in the competence assessment process, a practice that is consistently supported across clinical authorities. Finally, a good deal of research, including our own, has provided empirical evidence supporting the notion that functions associated with Understanding and Appreciation can vary independently of each other and are impaired by different factors.

Whether Appreciation is seen as a separate concept or as a part of Understanding, its application poses inherent difficulties in legal or clinical judgments about competence. Some patients may not believe what they are told about their disorder or its treatment, yet they may have objectively reasonable grounds for challenging their physicians' opinions.

> After fourteen prior hospitalizations for treatment of manic episodes, a 33-year-old man was again admitted to a psychiatric hospital. Since the onset of his disorder 6 years before, he had been tried on a large number of maintenance medications, none of which had prevented recurrence of mania. After stabilization of his acute condition, his current psychiatrist, who had

not treated him previously, approached him about using a new combination of medications after discharge. Each of the medications presented some risk of unpleasant side effects, but the psychiatrist was enthusiastic about their potential for reducing the frequency of recurrences of mania. Thus, she was taken aback by the patient's rejection of the proposal. "I don't believe any of these medications are going to help," he said. "Nothing has before and I don't see why this is going to be any different."

In contrast to the woman who denied that her toes were gangrenous, this patient's beliefs seem clearly rooted in his previous experience. Indeed, we might almost say that he is applying the scientific method to reach his conclusion. After multiple failures of new treatment regimens, he has learned to discount the enthusiasm of his physicians; he always seems to be the exception to their stories of therapeutic success. There appears to be a qualitative difference between his position and the denial of the patient with gangrene in the previous case example. It seems reasonable to deny her the right to make her own treatment decisions; after all, she is unable to acknowledge the reality of her condition. This patient, however, seems to appreciate all too well his own fragile state. We might want to reason with him — if we truly had a basis for believing that the new treatment regimen would make a difference — but we would have a hard time supporting the fairness of depriving him of the power of choice.

Because of cases like this, and others in which patients' beliefs are based on subcultural categorizations of illness and treatment, it is clear that mere disagreement with physicians' characterization of the situation is not an adequate basis for concluding that someone is incompetent. Rather, patients' nonacknowledgement of their illness or the relevant consequences of treatment options should be counted as a failure of Appreciation only when patients' choices are based on premises (beliefs) that meet several tests.

First, *the patient's belief must be substantially irrational, unrealistic, or a considerable distortion of reality*. Note that this point does not question patients' *choices*; it questions the irrational quality of the *beliefs or premises* on which their choices are based. Many of us might consider a particular choice to be deviant, in the sense that few people might select it under the circumstances. Yet the choice should not be considered to reflect a lack of Appreciation if it is based on premises that manifest no great irrationality. That seems true for the man with recurrent mania, as well as in the following case.

> A 67-year-old man with metastatic cancer of the prostate was faced with the question of whether to consent to aggressive chemotherapy that might extend his life 6 months to a year but would induce anorexia, nausea, vomiting, and probably require that he be bedridden during much of that time. He opted instead for a less aggressive approach that would probably lead to his much more rapid demise. But during much of his remaining time he would be able to live at home and do the things he enjoyed, including fishing. His choice was related to his belief that the most valuable thing in his life was his relationship with his grandchildren. He wanted most to have them remember him for the fishing outings they took with him every week.

In another case involving the same options and choice as in the case above, a different belief underlying the choice might make a considerable difference with regard to the questionable status of the patient's Appreciation. Were his choice for the shorter life course related to his belief that the world would end in 6 months, a date reached on the basis of a complex exercise in numerology, we might be more willing to question the patient's decision-making abilities.

The well-known story of Justice Robert Jackson of the United States Supreme Court illustrates the values involved here. Justice Jackson, an intellectual force on the Court in the late 1940s, was told after he suffered a heart attack that he had two choices. He could continue with the heavy workload that his position entailed, which would ensure a rapid demise, or he could retire from the Court, in which case he might live for many years. Like the patient with prostate cancer in our case example, Justice Jackson opted to continue doing what he loved — in this case, his work — even at the cost of his health. He died not long thereafter, having made the choice that seemed right to him. Of course, without evidence that his decision was based on irrational ideas or a serious distortion of reality, that choice was respected, as it should have been.

Second, *the belief must be the consequence of impaired cognition or affect.* Not all irrational or illogical beliefs can easily be dismissed as a lack of Appreciation. Most traditional religious beliefs are "irrational" in the sense that they do not and need not be justified by logical or empirical proof. In fact, one cannot automatically dismiss the numerologist's belief as constituting a lack of Appreciation regarding the consequences of choosing a shorter life span. To do so would, in principle, risk depriving patients of autonomous choice based on values — even if unpopular or eccentric — that they should have the freedom to use for guidance in their lives.

A special set of issues is raised by patients who offer religious beliefs as the justification for their challenge to physicians' views of their condition and treatment.

Seven years after an initial diagnosis of and surgery for breast cancer, a 43-year-old woman began having neck stiffness and tingling in her arm. A chiropractor took cervical spine films, which revealed a compression fracture, and a subsequent MRI showed multiple cervical spine metastases. At least one of the masses appeared to be impinging on the spinal cord. The nature of her problem was explained to her, including the possibility of quadriplegia, respiratory paralysis, and even death without rapid treatment. She was told that immediate treatment with intravenous steroids plus radiation therapy was likely to be effective over a period of days. Although she clearly understood what she was told, the patient declined any further medical treatment. She told a psychiatric consultant that she wanted to go home, because the power of faith was the best way to take care of her problem. Accepting any medical treatment would be giving in to fear and would interfere with the spiritual healing. Further probing revealed that the patient had, over the past several years, become

active in a religious group that emphasized the power of spiritual
healing and had consistently adhered to their doctrines.

Our usual criteria for assessing appreciation fail us here. Religious
beliefs are, by definition, neither rational nor irrational. Rationality,
one might say, is beside the point. Moreover, our society generally has
placed religious beliefs beyond the purview of the courts and other
administrative structures. In part, this relates to our reluctance to identify some religious beliefs as acceptable and others as not. And, since
freedom of belief is of little value without the freedom to act on one's
beliefs, we will usually permit competent adults to follow their religious convictions, even if that leads to harm. Only when the well-
being of minors or of other third parties is involved are the courts
likely to intervene.

Thus, when patients express religious bases for differing with their
physicians' appraisal of their situations, our inquiry is usually limited
to ascertaining that they are reflecting genuine religious beliefs. Among
the criteria useful for making such a determination are whether the
patient's beliefs predate the treatment decision, whether they are re-
flective of religious views held by others (i.e., not idiosyncratic to the
patient him- or herself), and whether the patient has previously be-
haved in ways consistent with these beliefs. The patient in our case
example meets these criteria. We might decide differently than she
did, but she is free to make her own choice.

Third, *the belief must be relevant to the patient's treatment decision.*
Strange beliefs or even psychotic delusions that do not enter into the
patient's reasons for deciding on a particular treatment are not relevant for Appreciation; the concept itself has no meaning outside the
decision-making process.

The instances of illogical belief about which law and ethics are
concerned are those in which patients' critical beliefs are directly related to mental disorder or cognitive impairment. To the extent that
patients' choices are based on distorted or irrational beliefs that are
part of a process of mental disorder or psychological dysfunction, their
choices presumably do not reflect the judgments that they would otherwise have made for themselves.

In subsequent chapters, we return often to these difficult matters of definition for Appreciation, because they tread on uneven ground that has many potential pitfalls. In some cases they require difficult judgments by clinicians, with potential for error that poses a risk of unwarranted deprivation of patients' autonomy. Yet judgments about the phenomena involved in lack of Appreciation cannot be ignored in clinical practice, for example, in cases like that of the woman with the gangrenous toes. To do so would fail to recognize that her adequate Understanding does not protect her from an "uninformed" decision (with potentially dangerous consequences) based on irrational denial of her illness.

Clinical Interpretation of the Concept

The inability that the law calls "failure of Appreciation" has long been identified in clinical practice by other terms and concepts. When clinicians encounter patients like the woman with the gangrenous toes, they refer to patients' misidentifications of their conditions, and of the consequences of their illnesses, as a "lack of insight" regarding their disorders. Clinicians also are accustomed to encountering patients whose "denial" impairs their ability to choose a course of action. Sometimes it is the illness that is denied, while at other times it is a denial of the probable consequences of treatment itself.

A few months following the death of her mother-in-law, a 54-year-old woman without previous psychiatric history became severely depressed. She expressed the belief, which was clearly disconfirmed by family members, that she gave her mother-in-law the wrong medication, and thus was responsible for her death. She also appeared to have delusions about the functioning of her gastrointestinal tract. Since she had multiple medical problems, her physicians had to proceed cautiously with the use of antidepressant medication, and she was not responding to the dosages she could tolerate. Meanwhile, her angina pectoris was getting worse and the cardiologists recommended immediate cardiac catheterization to see whether surgery was indicated.

The patient, however, refused. Probing her reasoning, it became clear that she was hopeless about the future, believing that nothing would make her better. She asked only to be allowed to go home, where she could lie in her own bed until she died. This, after all, was what she deserved, she said, since her negligence had been the cause of her mother-in-law's death.

As in this case, sometimes the patient's distorted belief is associated with delusional symptoms related to a major affective disorder. Lack of insight is also a common symptom of schizophrenia, and there are numerous investigations of its manifestation in a variety of patient groups (Appelbaum & Grisso, 1995). In our own studies of patients' Appreciation, we found that serious failure to acknowledge symptoms and diagnoses (as verified by assessments of newly admitted inpatients) was more common among patients with schizophrenia (about 35 percent) than among patients with major depression (5 percent). Rigid denial of the potential value of treatment was less common, being manifested by about 13 to 14 percent of patients in both of the groups with mental illnesses.

Denial and lack of insight, however, are best seen as psychological phenomena that occur on a continuum, not only in relation to major mental illnesses. Denial and distortion are psychological defenses, employed to some degree by all of us, most commonly in stressful circumstances. As such, these mechanisms can occur in adaptive and maladaptive forms.

In fact, frank denial or gross minimization of the nature of an obvious illness may be seen in many persons who present no evidence of major mental disorder. In our study, for example, questionable Appreciation of symptoms of heart disease was found in about 10 percent of patients with angina pectoris, none of whom manifested symptoms of major mental disorder. These are sometimes cases in which the person's psychological resources for dealing with the illness are fragile and therefore in danger of disintegration. Under such conditions, cognitive distortions sometimes become so great that patients' stated beliefs may contradict reality, even without delusional or affective disorder, and seriously interfere with their ability to weigh meaningfully the consequences of various treatment options.

Implications for Competence Assessment

The process of assessing Appreciation generally will involve an inquiry into patients' reasons for choosing a particular treatment option. That inquiry must involve an exploration of sufficient detail to determine the premises (beliefs) underlying the patient's reasoning. The woman with severe depression discussed above, for example, reasoned that her chances of death were similar with or without treatment. The premise or critical belief behind this reasoning was that God inexorably visits punishment on sinful people, and that she was especially sinful. We cannot comment on the accuracy of the former belief, but the latter seemed manifestly untrue and due to her profound depression.

Less pronounced depression, on the other hand, often presents considerable difficulties in competence assessment (Sullivan & Youngner, 1994). It is easy for caregivers to perceive patients' expressions of discouragement or hopelessness as reasonable reactions to patients' illnesses, when they may actually reflect their depressed moods. This "false empathy" can lead clinicians to accept decisions to forego treatment that are, in fact, of questionable competence. Since it is often impossible to know the extent to which depression is affecting patients' appreciation, evaluators need to have a high index of suspicion. The best course may be to defer a decision about patients' capacities (see Chapter 5), and about the proper course of treatment, while antidepressant medication is instituted on an empirical basis.

When patients' critical beliefs are illogical or irrational, it will be especially important to obtain information that can assist in interpreting the significance of those beliefs when applying the Appreciation requirement. As explained in the previous discussion of Appreciation as a competence concept, not all illogical beliefs contribute to a lack of Appreciation. They must be considered in the context of patients' clinical conditions, their history of mental disorder and typical style of adaptation to stress, and their religious and cultural background. Judgments about Appreciation are often difficult; proper assessment of the related questions is therefore essential to avoid error in our judgments that may unfairly deprive patients of their rights to autonomous choice and protection from choices made incompetently.

REASONING

> A 48-year-old woman with a chronic mental disorder of uncertain etiology became psychotically depressed. She told her psychiatrist that she was a prostitute who deserved to be "exterminated," and that was what they should do with her. When electroconvulsive therapy was recommended, she declined, saying that she already had brain damage and the procedure was likely to kill her. One of her physicians challenged her decision, asking why, if she wanted to die, she would turn down the opportunity to receive a treatment that she thought was likely to lead to that result. The patient offered no coherent response.

Reasoning as a Competence Concept

Even when patients have met the Understanding and Appreciation requirements (which the patient in this case example probably did not), courts and ethicists have sometimes recognized the need to examine whether they appear to be able to manipulate information rationally. The concern here is with patients' abilities to engage in logical *processes* when using the information that they understand and appreciate in arriving at a decision. We call this the *Reasoning* requirement for competence.

Difficulties in the processing of information to reach a decision can take several forms, which we examine next. Sometimes patients seem unable to deal with the complexity of the options; at other times, as in the example above, patients' choices seem not to follow from their stated preferences for various consequences. Some patients may also be overwhelmed by the decision-making task.

It is important to distinguish the Reasoning requirement from other issues with which it is often confused. Much of this confusion derives from the various ways that clinicians and courts have used the term "irrational" in describing patients' abilities to make treatment decisions.

Specifically, sometimes patients' decisions are said to be "irrational" because they are based on implausible presumptions about treatment consequences. This is close to our definition of Appreciation, and it refers to the *beliefs* that go into patients' decision-making tasks.

At other times patients' decisions are said to be "irrational" because there is something wrong with *the way they use information* to reach a decision. This is the focus of the Reasoning requirement, which pertains to potential irrationality in the *processing* of information, not in the *content* or propositions that are processed (which is the point of the Appreciation requirement). It is quite possible to process irrational beliefs logically, thereby fulfilling the Reasoning requirement while having poor Appreciation. And, of course, one can fully appreciate various consequences of treatment, yet have difficulties using those beliefs logically when combining information to reach a decision.

Yet another way in which the term "irrational" has been used in reference to competence to make treatment decisions has focused on the choice itself. The patient's actual choice, being considered by others as unconventional or not in the patient's best medical interest, is said to be irrational or unwise. Notice that this usage focuses on a normative judgment about the advisability of the *outcome* of the decision process, while the Reasoning requirement focuses on the *process.* It is quite possible for a logical reasoning process to lead to an unpopular or eccentric choice. As we noted in this chapter's introductory comments, a choice that is perceived by others as irrational in this sense should be respected — as long as Understanding, Appreciation, and Reasoning are intact — consistent with the value that society places on protecting its citizens' autonomy to choose for themselves.

As with Appreciation, we are concerned here with substantial impairments of Reasoning ability that arise from the effects of psychopathology or cognitive deficits. The Reasoning criterion is not appropriately used to deny decision-making power to people whose style of making choices deviates from some abstract norm of "rationality." Some people choose impulsively, preferring to avoid prolonged deliberation. Others "go with their gut," relying on emotional or intuitive factors to guide them in their decisions. It is their right to make choices as they please, so long as mental disorders or limitations on cognition do not prevent them from doing otherwise. The patient who elects to trust her physician's judgment, without a thorough inquiry into the risks and benefits of treatment, is making a competent choice. However, the patient who has no alternative but to rely on other people because she lacks the ability to weigh risks and benefits on her own may well not be a competent decision maker.

Clinical Interpretation of the Concept

The process of making practical decisions has been represented theoretically by cognitive psychologists in a number of problem-solving models (e.g., Goldfried & D'Zurilla, 1969; Hogarth, 1987; Janis & Mann, 1977; Spivack, Platt, & Shure, 1976). A composite of these models suggests the following way of thinking about the basic functions that are involved — or should be involved — when patients process information to reach a decision about treatment:

- *Problem Focus:* The decision maker needs to be able to stay focused on the problem of selecting a treatment. To the extent that other unrelated problems and concerns intrude, the decision-making process may deteriorate.
- *Considering Options:* One needs to take into account the range of available options while processing the decision. A narrow focus on one alternative, without giving any consideration to others, does not promote a meaningful process of choosing among options.
- *Considering and Imagining Consequences:* The decision maker needs to consider the consequences of the options. In an informed consent procedure for treatment decisions, this would include not only considering the medical benefits and risks/discom-

forts that have been disclosed, but also the patient's ability to imagine the practical consequences for his or her everyday life.

- *Assessing Likelihood of Consequences:* The decision maker needs to be able to think about consequences in terms of the likelihood (probability) that they will occur.
- *Evaluating Consequences:* One needs to weigh the desirability of various potential consequences, based on one's own subjective values.
- *Deliberating:* The decision maker needs to engage in a process of comparing and "working with" the relevant consequences, their likelihoods, and their desirabilities, in order to reach a decision.

When one considers even this simplified view of the problem-solving process, it is doubtful whether any of us is a paragon of effective decision making in everyday situations, much less in times of crisis. Indeed, much attention has been devoted in recent psychological research to documenting the many ways in which people deviate from a purely "rational" model of decision making. The role of emotions in decisional processes has been a particular focus of concern (DiMasio, 1994). The question in clinical judgments about decision-making capacity, though, is whether a patient's mental abilities are so impaired by illness or disability that even basic functioning with regard to these considerations is seriously and negatively influenced.

The multiple functions associated with problem solving mean that deficits in Reasoning may manifest themselves in a number of ways. In the case described at the beginning of this section involving the depressed woman who wanted to die, the Reasoning question was raised because the patient's choice simply did not follow from her own propositions (which themselves reflected defects in Appreciation). One listens to how the patient is weighting, positively and negatively, each of the consequences of options A, B, and C. Not questioning the wisdom of any of these consequential preferences, one considers what would be the logical choice given this patient's stated evaluation of the various consequences. When one does, it leads to option B; yet the patient has chosen option C. In other cases, patients may be unable to manage the range of information that the decision requires.

A man with mild mental retardation and a history of poor impulse control was faced with the question of whether to undergo a surgical procedure for chronic inflammatory bowel disease, to rely on his existing medical treatment, or to try a new medication regimen. Each of these options had different risks and benefits. In particular, surgery would have meant a period of hospitalization and subsequent bed rest which the patient had always found difficult to tolerate in the past. A careful and simplified disclosure process by the patient's attending gastroenterologist seemed to result in his understanding each of the consequences of the alternative treatments. He chose surgery. When asked how he arrived at this choice, the patient only talked about the surgical option, focusing on wanting to get the diseased portion of bowel out of his body. The physician tried to get him to compare two or three of the alternatives at once, but he became confused and retreated to talking only about the one he had chosen.

In cases such as this one, questions are raised concerning whether the patient has the capacity to weigh the consequences of several alternatives at once, a process that seems essential to making an informed choice. Other patients may be so overwhelmed by anxiety or emotion that they are unable — in the situation in which they find themselves — even to engage in a Reasoning process, although in other situations they might be unimpaired.

A 21-year-old woman in her 32nd week of pregnancy was admitted to an obstetrical service with preeclampsia. Her blood pressure was elevated, she had significant edema, and there were substantial amounts of protein in her urine, indicative of kidney failure. Treatment for the condition, which untreated presents the risks of stroke, seizures, and fetal and maternal death, involves delivery of the fetus. Afterwards, the symptoms generally resolve. All this was explained to the patient, and though she appeared to understand, she refused to permit induction of labor, because that would involve insertion of a small needle, of which she was terribly afraid. She had reportedly been afraid of needles all her life. When a psychiatric consultant was called to see her, her affect was described as "hysterical"; she was crying, screaming, and unable to sustain a conversation. After several failed attempts to talk with her, and even an unsuccessful effort to have her hypnotized, so that the needle could be inserted, the consultant decided that she was incompetent. An intravenous line was inserted involuntarily, and labor was induced. After a successful delivery, the patient indicated that she thought the treatment team had done the right thing.

People vary in their predispositions to anxiety and to emotional reactions that may limit their abilities to reason. Although stress and concomitant anxiety complicate many patients' decision making, for some, as for the patient in this case example, it can become crippling. At that point, especially when the stakes are high, they may be incompetent to make treatment decisions.

Some research has found deficits among inpatients with specific mental disorders in their abilities to process information during problem solving. But there have been many contradictory results, and often such studies have not focused on decisions related to treatment. Our own studies of patients' reasoning concerning treatment choices (Grisso & Appelbaum, 1995b) employed a measure designed to assess decision-making functions like those in the list above. We found that, as a group, patients with schizophrenia or major depression performed poorly more often than did their non-ill comparison groups. Nevertheless, many of the patients performed as well as their comparison subjects. This suggests that while diagnosis may be used to alert the clinician that there is a heightened risk of deficiencies in problem-solving abilities, diagnosis is not a good substitute for assessing the problem-solving abilities themselves.

Implications for Competence Assessment

There are few practical clinical methods for assessing patients' problem-solving capacities. Some aspects of cognitive ability related to these capacities are similar to functions assessed in mental status examinations or intelligence tests. In many cases, however, it will be difficult to make inferences about patients' abilities to reason about treatment decisions based on performance scores on more general indices of information processing.

Therefore, the assessment of patients' abilities related to the Reasoning requirement is best handled by an inquiry to patients after their treatment options have been disclosed to them. For example, they may be asked to "think aloud" as they work with the information to reach a decision, or they can be queried about their reasoning after they have stated a choice. As patients describe their reasoning, one can take stock of the degree to which they appear to consider the range of options, how they have weighted or evaluated the desirability of various consequences of these options, and whether their final choices appear to flow logically from their views of the consequences. More specific methods for doing this will be described in Chapters 5 and 6.

SUMMARY

In this chapter, we have identified and characterized the types of abilities that have been considered important — in law, ethics, and clinical practice — for assessing patients' competence to consent to treatment. We referred to these as ability requirements for competence to consent to treatment, and we identified four types of abilities:

1. *Expressing a Choice*, referring to the patient's ability to state a preference;
2. *Understanding*, referring to the ability to comprehend the information provided in the treatment disclosure for informed consent;
3. *Appreciation*, referring to the patient's beliefs about the disorder and potential treatments, especially the ability to apply realistically to one's own situation that which is understood; and
4. *Reasoning*, referring to the ability to process treatment information and one's preferences in a logical manner.

During the discussions, we noted several important things to remember when working with these concepts:

- One can expect courts to apply one or more of these abilities in
  judging competence to consent to treatment. Which ones are
  employed, however, will vary across courts in different jurisdictions. Clinicians should seek information from legal professionals
  in their own communities concerning the applicable requirements and their relation to the abilities we have described.

- Ethicists differ in their notions of the best way to conceptualize
  the critical abilities associated with competence to consent to
  treatment. Our way of organizing and defining the abilities attempts to capture concepts that have been recognized with some
  consensus as requiring attention in order to protect the autonomy
  and welfare of patients during treatment decision making.

- Although the ability concepts we have described are relevant for
  judgments about patients' competence, those judgments are not
  determined simply on the basis of deficits in these abilities. No
  particular level or type of deficit in ability is determinative in all
  cases. As we pointed out in Chapter 2, competence judgments
  must take into account clinical and situational information as
  well.

- The fact that a patient's choice seems unwise provides a basis for
  close examination of the patient's abilities for treatment decision
  making. It does not in itself, however, provide a basis for a finding of incompetence to decide.

- Patients with mental disorders and disabilities may, as a group, be
  at greater risk of manifesting deficits in the abilities described
  here. On the other hand, many members of this group do not
  display such impairments. The mere fact that a patient manifests
  mental disorder (either chronic or secondary to the current medical situation), mental retardation, or cognitive impairment should
  not create a presumption that the patient has deficits in the relevant abilities.

- Assessment of the abilities described here is best accomplished by
  combining an evaluation of the patient's clinical condition with a

direct assessment of the patient's actual understanding, appreciation, reasoning, and ability to express a choice within the context
of the present treatment situation.

Our description of the four abilities includes special attention to
identifying the conceptual differences between them. One might ask,
however, whether the abilities are really so different in an empirical
sense. For example, both Understanding and Reasoning can be influenced negatively by pathological mental conditions and in patients
with poorer general intellectual capacity. Therefore, one would have
good reason to suspect that these two abilities are correlated, and that
a patient who has deficits in one area might be expected to have
deficits in the other area. If this were true, one would want to take it
into account during assessment, perhaps avoiding the effort of evaluating more than one ability.

Our studies of mentally ill and medically ill patients have suggested
that patients' Understanding and Reasoning with treatment information are, indeed, substantially correlated (Grisso & Appelbaum,
1995a, b; Grisso, Appelbaum, Mulvey, & Fletcher, 1995). Yet we en-
countered some patients who performed poorly on Reasoning tasks
when they had performed adequately on Understanding tasks. Moreover, the relation of both of these abilities to Appreciation was far less
predictable.

In assessing individual clinical cases, therefore, we recommend that
when judgments of decision-making capacity (based on the applicable
criteria for competence in that jurisdiction) require knowledge of all
of these abilities, all of them should be assessed. Our experience suggests that there is not enough of a relation among these abilities to use
performance on one of them to support presumptions about patients'
status on the others.

Having discussed the doctrine of informed consent, maxims regarding competence to consent to treatment, and abilities that are conceptually associated with competence, we are now ready to approach the
assessment process itself. When and how should competence assessments be performed?

4

WHEN PATIENTS' DECISION MAKING SHOULD BE ASSESSED

Whether they recognize it or not, most clinicians assess their patients' decision-making abilities as part of every encounter. Ordinarily, this occurs unconsciously, as clinicians take notice of patients' dress, demeanor, communicative skills, intelligence, ability to attend to a conversation, apparent understanding, and ability to reach a decision. Since we all assume, appropriately, that the people with whom we deal are competent to make decisions about their own lives — indeed, the law makes a similar assumption — only when our unconscious monitoring detects something unexpected do we attend to it directly.

Thus, when the retired schoolteacher, who has always come to appointments with his internist immaculately dressed and groomed, appears in disheveled clothes with a 3-day growth of beard, the good clinician senses immediately that something is amiss. If an important decision about medical treatment needs to be made, the physician might well want to know more about the patient's condition before encouraging him to make a choice. An implicit process of monitoring the patient's decision-making capacities now becomes explicit. And, since more than intuition is involved, the clinician needs a strategy for performing this more detailed assessment.

This chapter highlights those circumstances in which clinicians may want to pay particular attention to patients' decision-making capacities, beyond the routine monitoring common to every therapeutic encounter. Such situations may arise in general medical or surgical treatment, psychiatric settings, or during the course of research with human subjects. We provide an overview of the clinical issues that are especially likely to provoke concern about patients' competence, along with data from research on decision-making abilities that identifies risk factors for impaired capacities of which clinicians should be aware.

ABRUPT CHANGES IN PATIENTS' MENTAL STATE

Perhaps the most self-evident circumstance calling for greater attention to patients' decision-making capacities is when there have been recent changes in patients' mental functioning. Patients may appear in their doctors' offices in a confused or disoriented condition. More subtle changes in mentation may be reflected in patients' behavior. A withdrawn patient suddenly becomes garrulous, or the jocular patient sullen. The natty dresser, as in the foregoing example, appears with clothes in disarray. Elderly patients are especially likely to show such changes, which often reflect alterations in their metabolic state, or can be due to fever, the side effects of medication, or even exhaustion.

> After many years of following a 76-year-old widow for her general medical problems, including hypertension and a congenital heart valve problem, her internist noted a change in her presentation in his office. Formerly lively and quick to joke with him, she seemed on her latest visit quiet and withdrawn. She had always been a bit on the suspicious side, but now that trait was heightened, as she questioned why he was prescribing an additional medication for her hypertension, why he needed to do an electrocardiogram (EKG), and on what basis he was recommending a referral to a cardiologist. His motives, she intimated, were related to the fees he would receive for the EKG and the kickback he would get from the cardiologist for referring her. She noted that in the last few days she had stopped taking her antihypertensives, because she didn't think she needed them

anymore, and wasn't sure what was in them anyway. Within a few days, the patient developed a full-blown paranoid psychosis, which turned out to be the harbinger of early Alzheimer's disease. A guardianship was obtained so that her son could make treatment decisions on her behalf.

Of course, most clinicians' first concern in such circumstances will not be with patients' competence. They will want to know what has upset patients' mental equilibrium, and especially whether there are treatable medical causes. But the search for causes and the initiation of treatment both require a patient who is competent to consent to these interventions. Thus, attention to patients' decision-making abilities is inescapable. We will consider in Chapters 5 and 6 how to conduct an evaluation of decisional capacities, and in Chapters 7 and 8 what might be done if patients' impairments compromise their ability to make medical decisions for themselves. At this point, suffice it to say that abrupt changes in mental state call for attention to whether patients are still able to make medical treatment decisions.

WHEN PATIENTS REFUSE TREATMENT

Merely because a patient refuses recommendations for evaluation or therapy does not mean that a patient lacks competence to decide about medical treatment. Admittedly, it is tempting for physicians and other health professionals to believe that the only reason a patient might reject their suggestions regarding optimal care is because that person lacks the mental abilities to recognize the proper course of action. But that is clearly not the case. Indeed, a fair proportion of the educational efforts regarding informed consent directed at physicians in the last 30 years have been devoted to undercutting the presumption that treatment refusal equates to incompetence on the part of the patient.

People have many legitimate reasons for rejecting their caregivers' recommendations. Sometimes the value they place on relief of symptoms or prolongation of life is simply different from the weight their physicians give these interests. Often patients' decisions are influenced by their experiences with side effects of medication or the aftermath of interventional procedures, issues that may be given less weight by health professionals who themselves have never experienced these complications of treatment. Patients may also have information of which their caregivers are unaware regarding past response to treatment or susceptibility to adverse outcomes. The doctrine of informed consent was developed precisely to allow patients to make choices on these and other bases that might differ from the decisions their physicians would make.

There are, however, at least two reasons why a patient's rejection of treatment might legitimately heighten clinicians' sensitivity to possible impairment of decision-making abilities. First, physicians usually try to recommend treatment that will minimize the impact of the patient's disorder. Declining to follow that recommendation raises the risks of an adverse outcome for the patient. Although patients may sometimes know more than their physicians do about what is best for them, often they do not. Their decisions may reflect misinformation, irrational biases, or the influence of other persons without extensive medical knowledge. In most circumstances, rejecting the treatment recommended by a physician is a riskier decision than agreeing to the proposal. If one of the goals of the competence requirement is to protect patients from bad outcomes, this would seem like a situation in which particular attention to patients' capacities might well be warranted. The more adverse the likely outcome, of course, the more carefully the question of the patient's competence should be considered.

The second justification for centering attention on refusals of treatment is the empirical reality that many patients who refuse treatment do so because of diminished decision-making capacities. To admit this is by no means to agree that every patient who differs with his or her physician is incompetent. But as we have seen in the case examples in the preceding chapters, intellectual impairment, attentional difficulties, anxiety, denial, delusions, dementia and other manifestations of psychopathology and impaired cognition can all lead patients to reject recommendations for treatment. Most clinicians are well aware of this tendency. One of the major reasons for consultation requests to psychiatry in most inpatient facilities is concern about the competence of patients who refuse treatment.

> The attending neurologist on an inpatient unit requested a psychiatric consultation on a 79-year-old woman who had been hit by a truck six months earlier. In the wake of the accident, she developed memory problems and gait abnormalities, which raised the suspicion that she might be suffering from normal pressure hydrocephalus. Computerized tomography was not definitive, so the patient's neurologist recommended a radioisotope study of her cerebrospinal fluid dynamics, a procedure involving injection of a small amount of isotope through a lumbar puncture. The patient refused, provoking the consultation request. On interview, she was pleasant but adamant about her refusal, saying that she would only change her mind if Dr. Lauren agreed. The consultant went off to find Dr. Lauren, until discussion with the staff on the unit revealed that he was a delusional figure invented by the patient. At times, she even talked about being married to Dr. Lauren. When the consultant suggested bringing in the patient's stepdaughter to talk with her, hoping she could persuade the patient to have the procedure, the patient indicated that her stepdaughter's opinion was of little consequence. She would only abide by Dr. Lauren's decision.

The importance of carefully examining the basis for a patient's rejection of treatment is obvious. Were this patient's refusal to have been taken at face value, with the assumption that she was making a competent choice, the delusions underlying her decision would never have been identified, and a potentially treatable condition left to worsen. Although persons concerned with patients' civil liberties often worry that physicians are too quick to request capacity evaluations when patients refuse treatment, studies in medical and surgical units suggest that most refusing patients are *not* referred for evaluation. This is true even when the risks of their decisions are substantial and there is good reason to believe that their mentation, and therefore their decisional abilities, may be impaired (Appelbaum & Roth, 1982).

A 55-year-old woman with hyperthyroidism was admitted to a surgical service for thyroidectomy. Almost immediately, the nurses noted that she was unable to stay in her bed, as ordered, or even in her room. She spent the day roaming the ward, wandering into the rooms of other patients, and asking loud and intrusive questions about their conditions. Her speech was pressured and there was an irritable quality to her interactions with other people. When a nurse's aide came to her room to collect a urine sample, the patient got into a shouting match with the woman, and demanded to be discharged from the hospital. The patient's sister arrived later that evening to take her home, and she was allowed to sign out without further evaluation.

The hypomanic behavior exhibited by this patient may have been the result of her hyperthyroid state, or may have reflected an underlying bipolar disorder. In either case, it raised serious questions about her ability to make a competent decision about leaving the hospital and foregoing surgery for what could become a life-threatening disorder. Here, the attending physician had too low a threshold for requesting a careful evaluation of the patient's decision-making capacities. The intent of the competence component of the doctrine of informed consent was thereby frustrated.

WHEN PATIENTS CONSENT TO TREATMENT THAT WILL BE ESPECIALLY INVASIVE OR RISKY

Critics of medical practices with regard to assessing competence sometimes assert that physicians are willing to overlook almost any degree of impairment if patients agree with their suggested course of treatment. Perhaps this generalization was once true, but if so, it no longer reflects many physicians' behavior. As knowledge has grown among health care professionals that patients lacking in decisional capacity cannot provide valid informed consents, physicians and others involved in patients' care increasingly have been willing to examine the competence even of patients who agree with their recommendations.

This is especially the case when patients have consented to unusually intrusive, experimental, or risky procedures. Examples might include bone marrow transplants, especially for genetic disorders that are not immediately life threatening; surgery to control seizure disorders by removing substantial amounts of brain tissue; and multiple organ transplants. Of course, within a few years, some of these procedures may become routine, replaced on the list by a new set of cutting-edge medical and surgical interventions, perhaps including gene therapy.

Is it reasonable to require formal assessments of functions related to competence whenever a patient undergoes an especially intrusive or innovative procedure? Evaluations of decision-making capacity carry costs of their own, including delay, expense, and a certain amount of inconvenience for patients. Centers performing procedures that fall into the categories we are discussing might well want to devise criteria by which to judge when decisional abilities require formal assessment. Some clinicians will want to use them routinely, perhaps as much for self-protective purposes — in the event their consent procedures are challenged — as to protect patients' interests. Even if patients' deficits are not so profound as ordinarily to warrant formal assessment of capacity, everyone involved in these cases may feel more comfortable being assured that patients are capable of making decisions. For both reasons, when dealing with the riskiest interventions, about which the least is known, routine use may indeed be reasonable. In other cases, however, the requirement for evaluation of decisional capacity could be limited to situations in which doubts exist about patients' decision making.

Similar considerations may apply in research with human subjects, particularly if the protocols involved offer little or no prospect of benefit to the participants. Recent controversies over the legitimacy of involving patients with schizophrenia and other psychotic disorders in projects that put them at risk for exacerbation of symptoms or relapse arose, in part, because of concern over whether the research subjects were able to make competent decisions about participation. Research on subjects with dementing disorders raises nearly identical issues. Although less often considered, many subjects of research involving severe medical disorders may also experience impaired capacities as a result of their illnesses.

As the ratio of risks to benefits from participation in research increases, and doubts about subjects' capacities grow, the rationale for routine screening of the capacities of research subjects becomes more persuasive. Institutional review boards (IRBs), which oversee research in most facilities, only rarely have exercised their powers to require investigators to undertake such efforts. The availability of structured instruments suitable for screening purposes, such as the one discussed in Chapter 6, may make investigators and IRBs alike more willing to consider regular screening of subjects in high risk research, especially when their capacities may be called into question.

WHEN PATIENTS DISPLAY ONE OR MORE RISK FACTORS FOR IMPAIRED DECISION MAKING

The presence of factors that may elevate the risk of impaired decision making is never determinative of incompetence. Nonetheless, knowledge of such factors may help clinicians and policy makers target particular populations for routine screening or extra care in assessment. There are only a relatively small number of studies on which we can draw to identify variables that increase the risk that patients may be incompetent. Fortunately, these studies are supplemented by a good deal of clinical experience. Because the task here is only to characterize patients who may require more careful evaluation — rather than to identify one group or another as incapable of making meaningful decisions — both bodies of data, albeit imperfect, can be helpful.

Diagnosis

As we discussed in Chapter 2, no diagnosis carries with it a conclusive presumption of a patient's incompetence. That was not always the case. Prior to the last generation, patients diagnosed as psychotic, mentally retarded, or demented often lost their decision-making powers as a matter of course, with little or no inquiry into their actual functioning. The situation changed as clinicians recognized that many patients with severe mental disorders such as schizophrenia, with mild to moderate dementia, and with serious medical illnesses that can alter mentation nonetheless have adequate capacities to make decisions about their medical care. Evolving along with clinical understanding, the law too now recognizes that a particularized inquiry is required into patients' actual decision-making capacity before they are stripped of their decisional rights.

One week after a mass that was thought to be malignant was discovered in her breast, a 51-year-old woman with a history of 25 years of outpatient treatment for chronic schizophrenia became suicidal and experienced her first psychiatric hospitalization. Usually, the next step in the workup would have been to biopsy the mass, but the patient was unwilling to consent to the procedure. Instead, she asked to be discharged from the hospital so she could go home to pray, pay her bills, and take care of her home. This decision seemed unreasonable to her caregivers, who questioned her competence and requested a psychiatric assessment of her decision-making capacities. The consultant found that she understood the information communicated to her and appreciated the situation and its likely consequences. Moreover, she maintained that she was willing to accept treatment, albeit not immediately. She promised that the day after discharge she would call the surgeon to schedule the biopsy. The consultant viewed the request for discharge as an attempt to reestablish control over her life, which had been shattered by the diagnosis of probable malignancy and by her hospitalization. Because her decisional abilities appeared to be intact, he recommended allowing the patient to leave the hospital and to deal with the biopsy as she had proposed. The patient kept her promise to call the surgeon immediately after discharge, had a biopsy the following week, and underwent a definitive procedure to remove the mass a few weeks later.

It was not unreasonable for the attending physician in this case to request a detailed evaluation of the patient's decision making, since her diagnosis put her in a group at higher risk of impairment. Moreover, her choice was somewhat unusual, since most women in her situation proceed to biopsy immediately. Nonetheless, careful assessment showed that her decision was based on a full understanding of her situation and an appreciation of its potential consequences, and was reached by rational thought processes. The same will be true for many patients with high risk diagnoses.

Which diagnostic groups are at increased risk of decisional incapacity? Most clinicians would point first to patients with dementia, delirium, or other forms of organic impairment. Studies of psychiatric consultations to evaluate patients' decision-making abilities show consistently that organic brain syndromes are overrepresented among patients found to lack capacity compared with those thought to be able to make their own medical decisions. Moreover, when patients with dementia are compared directly with similar aged controls, they perform significantly worse on all of the major standards for the assessment of decision-making capacity. Even among the demented group, however, there is considerable variation in capacity. One major study suggested that impairment in word fluency and attentional abilities best differentiate capable from incapable patients with dementia (Marson, Ingram, Cody, & Harrell, 1995).

Mental illness is undoubtedly the next diagnostic category at which most clinicians would look to find persons at increased risk of incompetence. But mental illnesses are heterogeneous, with varied impact on cognition. Our studies, which contrasted the decision-making of patients with schizophrenia, major depression, and ischemic heart disease with non-ill community-based comparison groups, found that schizophrenia was associated with a significant increase in levels of decisional impairment (Grisso & Appelbaum, 1995b). This is a finding that has appeared consistently in other groups' studies as well. Among schizophrenic patients, however, there is considerable heterogeneity, partly due to variations in the severity of the symptoms associated with the disorder. Thus, in our study, those with high ratings of thought disorder and delusional thinking did significantly worse than their fellows with lower levels of these symptoms. Several studies have also shown that lower IQ correlates with poorer performance on competence-related measures in schizophrenia.

Depressed patients represent the other group of persons with mental illness whose decision-making capacities have been subject to systematic examination. Interestingly, the results are somewhat variable from study to study. Our work has shown that patients with major depression do significantly worse than matched controls on measures of understanding and reasoning, and that they display a higher rate of failure to appreciate the potential for treatment of their disorder compared with medical patients. Other studies have found modest decrements in reasoning ability and appreciation of their condition, while yet other work turned up no difference in performance between depressed and nondepressed patients. How can we account for these discrepancies? Common sense suggests we may be dealing with subjects with different degrees of depression, with those more seriously impaired doing worse. That assumption, however, has not been validated by the existing research. Resolution of this conundrum awaits further study.

The relationship between serious medical illness and decision-making difficulties has been all but unexplored. Several studies point to significant degrees of impairment among patients in intensive care units, which is hardly surprising. As noted above, we looked at the performance of hospitalized patients with ischemic heart disease, a potentially life-threatening condition. Despite their illness and the accompanying stress, these patients did no worse than matched community controls on tests of decision-making abilities. Of course, diagnoses that directly affect mental status, or that involve treatments that may impair mentation, are likely to have a more substantial impact on decisional capacity.

Other Clinical Factors

Regardless of diagnosis, there are other clinical variables that may place patients in a high risk group for impaired decision making. Psychopathological symptoms — even when insufficient to warrant a formal diagnosis of mental disorder—are such a variable. As patients become more anxious, for example, they are less able to attend to disclosures, process information, and reason about their options. The additive effects of anxiety, depression, and other symptoms of psychopathology can lead to impairment in cases in which any one category of symptom would not have had such an effect. Thus, composite measures of psychopathology, like the Brief Psychiatric Rating Scale, have been shown in many (although not all) studies to correlate with multiple measures of decision-making ability. The variation in results across studies, however, suggests that global psychopathology is, at best, only a rough indicator of inability to make medical treatment decisions.

Because gross impairment of cognitive functions, such as in dementia, is strongly related to problems in decisional function, one might expect that lesser degrees of cognitive difficulty would also predispose patients to a greater likelihood of incapacity. This may be especially true in elderly patients, even those without noticeable early signs of dementia, and in patients with mental retardation. Several studies have shown that the Mini-Mental State Examination (MMSE), a measure of cognitive impairment, predicts difficulties in treatment decision making among the elderly (e.g., Janofsky, McCarthy, & Folstein, 1992). In addition, clinical reports have suggested that frontal lobe dysfunction, which may be detected by neuropsychological testing or difficulty in performing executive functions, may impair the ability of patients to reason about their treatment. The impairment in these patients may be quite subtle, as they retain good abilities to comprehend information and interact socially with other people. A handful of efforts to correlate other neuropsychological functions with decision-making ability in a variety of diagnostic groups, however, have thus far come to naught.

After being found wandering the halls of the residence for the elderly where he lived, talking vaguely of suicide, a 76-year-old man was admitted to a psychiatric facility. He did well on treatment with antidepressants and low doses of an antipsychotic drug. As time for discharge approached, however, he turned down all options for group living, saying that he preferred to move in with a friend. The patient, however, had not seen the friend for two years and could not remember his name. The only other option he could suggest was moving into a hotel. When the hospital attorney was called to see him, he found the patient pleasant and socially appropriate, but firmly reiterating his determination to live with his friend. A psychiatric consultant, though, was impressed that the man could not remember his address or his doctor's name. By the end of the conversation, the patient had forgotten why the consultant had come to see him, saying that it had something to do with helping him to buy a house to live in. His speech was sprinkled with paraphasias, and he often had difficulty with word finding. Confronted with these results, and the impression that the patient failed to appreciate the consequences of his decision, the patient's lawyer talked him into accepting discharge to a group residential setting.

Treatment with some classes of medications, especially in the elderly, may also increase the risk of decisional impairment. Psychotropic medications in general, including antipsychotic medications, antianxiety agents (often used as hypnotics), and antidepressants, can diminish attention and the ability to process information. Indeed, many commonly used medications in other classes, including antihypertensives, histamine receptor blockers, and corticosteroids, can also affect mentation. Polypharmacy, which is all too frequent among hospitalized patients, and even among outpatients, compounds this problem, which may be especially profound in patients whose mental functioning is already marginal because of preclinical dementia, metabolic imbalances, and the stress of illness and hospitalization.

Situational Factors

Whether in hospitals or in ambulatory facilities, patients are often confronted with circumstances that make it more difficult for them to make decisions about their treatment. Because we know that high levels of anxiety impair decision making, we might hope that medical treatment settings would be designed to minimize the anxiety that patients feel. In fact, just the opposite often seems to be true. The threat to patients' health and well-being is, of course, frequently sufficient in itself to make them exceedingly fearful. Compounding that feeling, though, are the strange surroundings, unfamiliar language, lack of privacy, and intrusive questioning that seem to be part and parcel of the medical setting. The prospect of physical pain associated with diagnostic and treatment procedures exacerbates the situation.

These anxiety-provoking aspects of the hospital, clinic, and physician's office are multiplied many times for persons who have to deal with cultural differences as well. Immigrants, members of minority groups, working class patients, and those from isolated rural areas are often burdened both by difficulties with language and by the unfamiliar culture around them. This cultural mismatch may account, in part, for the finding in several studies of negative correlations between socioeconomic status or education and competence-related functions. Although inability to understand the sophisticated language and concepts used in medical settings undoubtedly plays a role here, the anxiety associated with being immersed in an alien and sometimes hostile-seeming environment cannot be ignored.

Another cultural factor that may impact patients' decision making is worth commenting on here, even though it may not reduce their decisional capacity *per se*. Patients from other cultures or from subcultural groups within our own society often have shared understandings of medical problems that do not correspond to those of modern medicine. Thus, some groups still cling to a concept of illness with which Galen would have been familiar, attributing disorder to an imbalance of bodily humors. Patients from these groups have not necessarily been exposed to theories of illness and its treatment that physicians might take for granted in dealing with upper middle-class patients born in the United States. Offering them such information can be an important part of the informed consent process. Once this information is provided, of course, patients may still choose a course of treatment consistent with their cultural beliefs. Yet, without such data, patients holding only subcultural theories of illness — even if competent — may not be able to make fully informed choices about their care.

A final situational factor is peculiar to patients hospitalized for treatment of mental disorder. In recent decades, the majority of patients admitted for psychiatric care have signed themselves into the hospital voluntarily. A significant fraction, however, is involuntarily committed. The differences between voluntary and involuntary patients vary across jurisdictions, depending on how the law defines who is eligible for inclusion in either group. Some studies have suggested that involuntary patients are less likely to be capable of making their own decisions. In particular, they seem to have higher rates of impaired appreciation of the fact that they are ill (which may be why hospitalization was carried out on an involuntary basis). Jurisdictions that blur the distinctions between the two groups, as by requiring that all patients be offered the opportunity to sign in voluntarily, even if only to avoid involuntary commitment, tend not to show this effect.

Age

A relationship between age and decision-making ability exists at both ends of the age spectrum. Since the incidence of dementia increases with age, older people, especially the "old old" (i.e., those older than 85 years of age) show increased rates of decisional impairment. Moreover, the elderly are more susceptible to the combined effects of anxiety, medication, and other risk factors. It should be stressed, however, that age *per se*, in the absence of cognitive impairment or other factors affecting capacity, does not reduce competence. Indeed, state statutes that once listed age in itself as a basis for the declaration of incapacity and the appointment of a guardian have been amended in the last few decades to avoid this implication.

At the younger end of the developmental time line, the acceptability of decision making by children and adolescents is governed by both statutory rules and medical practices. Minors generally are not legally entitled to make decisions for themselves; their parents or others standing *in loco parentis* have that power. The age of majority differs somewhat from state to state, usually varying between 16 and 18. There are exceptions in most states for emancipated minors (i.e., those who have been substantially responsible for their own care), minors who are themselves parents, and members of the armed forces.

In addition, state law often sets the age of decisional power somewhat lower for particular medical interventions, including mental health care, drug and alcohol abuse treatment, and family planning services. Adolescents as young as 12 years old may be able to make these decisions, although more typically the law sets the limit at 14 or 16 years of age.

How well are adolescents able to function when given the power to do so? An impressive body of research suggests that adolescents 14 years old and older tend to make decisions very much like those that would be made by adults (for one of the leading studies, see Weithorn and Campbell, 1982). Many health care professionals, recognizing the importance of these data, have taken to involving adolescents in treatment decisions. Treatment still cannot take place without the authorization of a parent or guardian, but these clinicians will refrain from treating adolescents who object to the intervention, even when parental consent has been obtained. Some questions remain, however, about the ability of many adolescents to put their decisions in the context of a future they may have difficulty anticipating. This question of "future orientation" is not usually considered relevant in assessing the competence of adults but may have a unique role to play where the issue is whether to respect the decision made by an adolescent.

SUMMARY

We have described four circumstances that can alert clinicians to the need for an evaluation of patients' decision-making capacities: abrupt changes in patients' mental states, patients' refusal of recommended treatment, patients' consent to especially invasive or risky treatment, and the presence of one or more risk factors to impaired decision making. Having considered these situations, we are now ready to address how competence evaluations can be performed. Chapter 5 covers issues relevant to competence evaluations in general, and Chapter 6 provides a look at one approach to structured assessment of patients' decision making using an instrument derived from our research.

5

ASSESSING PATIENTS' CAPACITIES TO CONSENT TO TREATMENT

In Chapter 4 we considered those circumstances in which a clinician might want to assess a patient's capacities to consent to treatment. Here we describe how that assessment should be performed, including (1) who should undertake the task, (2) the components, and (3) steps that can be taken to improve patients' performance.

WHO SHOULD PERFORM THE ASSESSMENT OF DECISION-MAKING CAPACITIES?

As we noted in Chapter 4, most clinicians perform intuitive assessments of patients' capacities during routine clinical interactions. Nurses and nursing aides who have regular contact with patients also have a role to play in identifying and raising with physicians questions of patients' decision-making capacities.

Once doubts arise about a patient's abilities to make decisions, the treating clinician will often be the person best situated to conduct a more extended evaluation of the patient's capacities. The special skills needed for this evaluation make it undesirable for the physician to delegate the evaluation task to nursing staff. In addition, seeking the assistance of an outside consultant should not necessarily be the immediate response when the question of competence first arises. Because the treating clinician is already with the patient, the physician's own evaluation can be performed without added delay or expense. In addition, the treating clinician is familiar with the patient's history and current condition, obviating the need to communicate this information to a consultant. And, not unimportantly, the patient will ordinarily have established with the clinician the kind of rapport required for an assessment of decisional capacity.

Given these advantages, there is no reason why a well-prepared attending physician cannot assess a patient's decisional capacities. Most hospitals' rules permit attending physicians to do so, and the courts have been equally receptive to evaluations performed by treating clinicians as to those conducted by psychiatrists or other consultants. But any clinician undertaking a formal assessment of a patient's capacities needs to be prepared for the task. This preparation includes acquiring a base of knowledge regarding the ethical, legal, and clinical underpinnings of the assessment of decisional capacities.

With regard to the ethical basis for the rules governing decisional competence, evaluators must be clear on the reasons why our society favors individual choice, even when that may result in less than optimal decisions from a medical perspective, and on the very limited grounds that we accept for abrogating such choice. Moreover, they need to keep in mind our strong societal presumption that persons are competent to make decisions for themselves unless convincing evidence is presented to the contrary. This assures that the assessment will be conducted in a manner that comports with the predilection of Western societies for maintaining patients' decisional autonomy.

Because the rules governing patients' decision-making rights are based in law, the evaluator must also be aware of the legal standards that govern competence determinations. As we discussed in Chapter 3, almost all jurisdictions base their rules on one or more of the four common components of competence standards: Expressing a Choice, Understanding, Appreciation, and Reasoning. Because, as we will review in detail in Chapter 7, one of the goals of an assessment is to approximate the decision that would be made by a court—if a judge were to review the case—the evaluating clinician needs also to be cognizant of the cutoffs commonly employed by the courts to determine how impaired patients must be before they will be declared incompetent to make treatment decisions.

Finally, from the clinical perspective, an assessment of decisional capacities is, at its core, an evaluation of a patient's mental functioning. Thus, the examiner must be comfortable with obtaining a psychiatric history and performing a general mental status evaluation, focusing specifically on those functions relevant to decision making. These include assessment of the patient's attention, mood, thinking (both form and structure), memory, and intellectual functioning.

These are not a daunting set of criteria, and there is no reason why most clinicians who make some effort to familiarize themselves with the relevant information cannot assess their own patients' decisional capacities. Indeed, apart from teaching the mental status examination, for which other references are available (e.g., Rogers, 1995; Shea, 1988), this book is designed precisely to allow them to do so.

There may, however, be reasons why it is preferable in particular cases to call for consultation regarding patients' capacities. Attending physicians may not have the basic knowledge to perform these evaluations, or may lack the time to spend on an assessment. Because a conclusion that a patient is not capable of making a treatment decision may set up an adversarial situation, especially if the patient contests the finding, treating clinicians may choose to avoid this threat to their relationship with the patient, preferring to let the consultant be the "bad guy." And, in particularly difficult cases, or where the risks of reaching the wrong conclusions about patients' capacities are especially high, there may be good reason to call in an expert who routinely performs evaluations of decisional capacity, if only to confirm the treating clinician's judgment.

Consultants who perform these assessments, of course, also should be aware of the ethical, legal, and clinical issues just discussed. Psychiatric or psychological expertise *per se* is no substitute for this specialized knowledge. In addition, an outside consultant must be sufficiently familiar with the relevant aspects of a patient's medical condition and treatment to allow discussion of these issues with the patient. Diagnosing the condition underlying a patient's mental impairment may also be required, along with knowledge of appropriate interventions.

In some facilities, formal assessments of patients' decision-making capacities are undertaken by multidisciplinary teams, ranging in size from two to six members. The teams may include clinicians, mental health professionals, bioethicists, and attorneys, in a variety of combinations. Although the maxim that two (or more) minds are better than one is often accurate, as yet there have been no comparisons of multidisciplinary teams with more traditional approaches to assessment. An important countervailing consideration is the cost and time involved in assembling these teams. At this point, it seems likely that their use will be restricted for the foreseeable future to academic centers, where they also serve training and research functions.

CONDUCTING THE ASSESSMENT

As experience with assessments of decisional capacity has accumulated, the steps that should be part of a valid examination have become better defined. Consultants called to assess a patient's decisional capacity must begin with some preliminary steps that attending physicians familiar with the case can avoid. Although we describe the steps involved in the usual chronological order, there will be times when it may make sense to alter the sequence to accommodate the clinical situation.

Ascertaining the Reasons for the Evaluation Request

It may seem self-evident that an evaluation of decisional capacity by a person not previously involved in the case requires some knowledge of why concerns have arisen about a patient's capacities. Consultation requests, however, often arrive devoid of this information. A psychiatric consultation service will frequently receive a consult form with nothing more on it than the words, "Please evaluate this patient's competence." There are several reasons why this is an inadequate basis on which to conduct the assessment requested.

First, whether or not a patient has adequate capacity to make a decision about treatment depends, in part, on the decisional demands that the patient faces (see Chapter 2). Decisions about a set of complex options for treatment that require trading off risks and benefits call for a level of functioning well beyond what may be needed for decisions in which the medical options are straightforward and limited. Thus, the consultant needs to know something about the patient's medical situation and the options with which the patient is faced.

Second, an additional determinant of whether patients would be judged legally competent to make treatment decisions relates to the consequences of their choices (see Chapter 2). As the potential for an adverse outcome rises, the courts — supported by many ethicists — tend to require less evidence of impairment before depriving patients of the power to make their own decisions. Without some sense of the options that patients have and the consequences of those options, an evaluator has no way of factoring these considerations into the assessment.

Third, a description of what provoked the consultation request will often contain important clues for the evaluator. Was the patient simply unresponsive when the attending physician approached him or her for a discussion about treatment? Did the patient appear to be confused about the information that was presented? Is the patient offering bizarre alternatives to the proposed treatment, or expressing concerns about the motives of people involved in the patient's care? Each of these possibilities suggests different underlying problems and a distinct orientation to the evaluation. Not knowing this information leaves the evaluator at a clear disadvantage.

Finally, paradoxical though it sounds, many consultation requests for evaluation of a patient's capacities are really not based on concerns about decisional competence at all. Attending physicians sometimes ask for competence assessments hoping that the consultant will talk the patient — whom they know to be competent — into accepting a treatment regimen that the patient is resisting. Conflict between patients and treatment staff can also become transmuted into a consultation for assessment of competence, when the real question behind the request is, "How on earth can we manage this impossible patient?" And it is not unheard of for an evaluation of competence to be requested as a way of "punishing" recalcitrant patients, as if to say, "We think you're crazy," or to frighten them with the possibility of losing control over their care. Even family members' personal and inap-

propriate motivations may be behind some requests for evaluations of
patients' treatment decision-making capacities: for example, their hope
that the evaluation will provide a tool that they can use in settling an
entirely different legal issue, such as whether the patient had the capacity to make a will with provisions they dislike. When any of these
motives underlies a consultation request, the evaluator who focuses
narrowly on a patient's decisional capacities is barking up the wrong
tree.

It is preferable, therefore, for a consultant who has been asked to
assess a patient's capacities to begin by speaking directly with the attending physician. (In some teaching hospitals, the resident in charge
of the case may actually be the most knowledgeable party.) Among the
questions that should be asked are these:

- Why is this consultation being requested?
- What evidence makes you think the patient may not be compe-
  tent to consent to treatment?
- What is the patient's current medical condition and what are the
  treatment choices with which the patient is faced?
- How is the patient responding to your suggestions for treatment?
- What factors do you think may be contributing to the problems
  that the patient is having in making a competent decision?

When the attending physician (or a suitable substitute) is unavail-
able or not forthcoming, the answers to some of these questions may
be obtained from a review of the patient's chart. Informants on an
inpatient unit, particularly the nurses involved in the patient's care,
can often provide an invaluable perspective on these issues as well.
But it is rarely desirable to proceed with an assessment of decisional
capacity without first discussing these issues with a physician directly
involved in the patient's care.

Preparing the Patient for the Evaluation

Two preliminary issues need to be addressed with a patient before the
evaluation itself can take place, regardless of whether the attending

physician or a consultant conducts it. Patients should, first of all, be told the nature and purpose of the evaluation. Informing patients of the purpose of the assessment that is about to begin alerts them to the importance of their performing as best they can. It also puts them on notice, as a matter of simple fairness, that their decision-making powers may be subject to challenge. Moreover, because most patients are perceptive enough to know that doctors do not stop by just for a chat, and are likely to be suspicious about the questions being asked, being open with patients reduces the risk of alienating them further.

Of course, when patients are told why their attending physician wants to talk with them, or that the examiner is a psychiatrist, psychologist, or other consultant who is here because, "Some of the people involved in your care have concerns about how well you are able to make decisions about your treatment," there are patients who will decline to proceed with the interview. Although that complicates the assessment (as we will see in Chapter 7), patients have the right to decide with whom they choose to speak. This is consistent with the rules of informed consent that apply in medicine more generally. And, as elsewhere in medicine, experienced examiners usually find that their openness actually facilitates the establishment of rapport with the patient.

Inevitably, the question arises as to whether a person who is suspected of being incompetent must give an informed consent to this kind of evaluation. We believe that the proper response is that when patients come for medical care — whether inpatient or outpatient — they or their appropriate surrogates consent at the outset to the performance of routine, non-invasive procedures that are part of that care. Thus, informed consent is not routinely obtained from patients every time a physical examination is performed or their blood pressure is taken, although patients are told in advance about what is being done and retain the power to refuse to cooperate. An assessment of decision-making capacity, if required, is similarly an intrinsic part of patient care, about which patients should be informed, but for which a discrete consent process is not required.

The second preliminary step before commencing the evaluation is to make certain that the patient has had an adequate opportunity to learn about his or her medical situation and the options for treatment. It is not possible to evaluate the competence of patients who have never been told about the considerations that may affect their care, or to whom the information has been presented in a confusing or contradictory fashion. The best way to accomplish this task is for the treating clinician, whether or not a consultant is involved, to go over with the patient the information relevant to a decision about treatment. This includes the nature of the patient's condition, the nature and purpose of the proposed treatment, its benefits and risks, and the alternative approaches, along with their benefits and risks. All too often it turns out that patients' apparent confusion or seemingly irrational rejection of treatment is due to their never having received an adequate disclosure of the information relevant to their care.

When a consultant is involved, there are numerous advantages to having the consultant present as this disclosure takes place. The consultant can assess the completeness of the disclosure, even interjecting questions to encourage the attending physician to flesh out the account. If the wording is too complex, the consultant can rephrase it, with the treating physician's concurrence regarding the accuracy of the reformulation, until it is clear that the patient understands. Observing the interaction also allows the consultant to gauge the patient's ability to attend to the disclosure, and the questions the patient asks (or fails to) can provide important data regarding the patient's state of mind.

Sometimes, unfortunately, when a consultation has been requested, the attending physician will not be available to accompany the consultant to see the patient. Even a resident with knowledge of the case may not be at hand. In those instances, there is no alternative but for the consultant to review with the patient that information relevant to the treatment decision. Here is where the consultant's understanding of the patient's medical condition is crucial. Whether obtained by direct discussion with the treatment team, a review of the patient's chart, or both, the evaluator must learn enough about the patient's situation to present a reasonable informed consent disclosure. The information disclosed to the patient will then form the basis for the subsequent assessment. If the evaluator feels unable to play this role, the consultation should be postponed until a physician sufficiently familiar with the case is available.

Conducting the Evaluation of the Patient's Abilities to Make Treatment Decisions

Once the patient has been adequately informed, the examiner can proceed with assessment of the relevant decision-making abilities. In most jurisdictions, this will involve an evaluation of one or more of the four standards for competence outlined in Chapter 3. When in doubt about the applicable standards, it is reasonable for the evaluator to gather data regarding the patient's functioning on all four standards, so that the maximum amount of information is available for the subsequent decision about the patient's capacities, after the operative standard is clarified.

Two general approaches can be taken to the assessment of capacities: a clinical interview or the use of a structured assessment tool. This chapter centers on the clinical interview in the evaluation process, but it is worth noting that a number of structured assessment tools have become available in the last few years. Almost all, however, have focused on a single type of medical decision (e.g., use of an advance directive [Janofsky, McCarthy, & Folstein, 1992], or treatment with electroconvulsive therapy [Bean, Nishisato, Rector, & Glancy, 1994]) or have been designed for use with a particular patient population (e.g., patients with Alzheimer's disease [Marson, Ingram, Cody, & Harrell, 1995]). Some data on the validity and reliability of these instruments are available, but their utility is limited by the treatments or populations for which they have been designed. Chapter 6 will assess the tool that we have developed — the MacArthur Competence Assessment Tool (or MacCAT) — which, to our knowledge, is the only instrument designed with sufficient flexibility to allow its use with cooperative patients regardless of the clinical situation.

Although clinical interviews do not use standardized questions and formal scoring criteria, they should not be entirely unstructured either. Evaluators should approach the patient with the relevant criteria in mind, and a plan for their systematic assessment. The following sections contain questions that may be helpful starting points in the assessment of each of the standards.

Ability to express a choice. This is the simplest standard, focused on the question of whether the patient can make and express a choice, and hold it with a reasonable degree of stability. Because many evaluations of decision-making capacity are prompted by a patient's refusal of treatment, and less often by a presumptively incompetent consent, this baseline ability will only rarely be at issue in the evaluation.

Suggested Questions

- "Have you decided whether to go along with your doctor's suggestions for treatment?"
- "Can you tell me what your decision is?" [Can be repeated at the end of the interview to assess stability of choice.]

Communication does not have to be verbal, of course, to be intelligible. Patients who are on respirators or impaired by strokes may still be able to communicate using hand signals, letter boards, eye blinks, and the like. When evaluators are dealing with such patients, the evaluators usually will need to frame their questions in a "yes–no" or multiple choice format. This is relatively easy for assessment of ability to express a choice itself. Determining how well patients understand information can also be successfully addressed by multiple-choice questions. Assessing Appreciation and Reasoning, however, are more difficult in this context. When the results of such an evaluation are significantly incomplete, the usual rules for determining whether patients are competent may have to be slightly modified. We will discuss this process in Chapter 7.

Ability to understand relevant information. The key here is whether the patient can assimilate the information required to be disclosed under the doctrine of informed consent. Patients should be encouraged to paraphrase the information that was presented to them, rather than spewing it back in precisely the same words. This helps to ensure that more than a simple input-output loop is involved.

Suggested Question

- "Please tell me in your own words what your doctor [or what I] told you about:
  ○ The nature of your condition.
  ○ The recommended treatment (or diagnostic test).
  ○ The possible benefits from the treatment.
  ○ The possible risks (or discomforts) of the treatment.
  ○ The possible risks and benefits of alternative treatments.
  ○ The possible risks and benefits of no treatment at all."

If the patient has trouble remembering the information that was presented, the examiner can redisclose the data in smaller pieces, questioning the patient after each segment to see if understanding has been attained.

Because risk information is, in many ways, among the most important data for the patient to grasp, further questioning may be warranted regarding the patient's understanding of the likelihood that a risk will materialize.

Suggested Question

- "Your doctor [or I] told you of a [percentage] chance that [named risk] might occur with treatment. In your own words, how likely to do you think the occurrence of [named risk] might be?"

It is also often useful to determine whether patients understand why the information is being given to them and the role that they are expected to play in the treatment decision. Patients who are puzzled about these issues may be less likely to attend to the disclosure or to know what to do with the information once they have it.

Suggested Questions

- "Why is your doctor [or the treatment team, or why am I] giving you all this information?
- What role do[es] he/she/we expect you to play in deciding whether you receive treatment?
- What will happen if you decide not to go along with your doctor's recommendation?"

Ability to appreciate the situation and its consequences. Appreciation relates to the patient's ability to apply the information abstractly understood to his or her own situation. Put differently, it concerns matters of belief rather than knowledge. The two prime areas of focus are patients' beliefs about whether or not they are ill, and about the likely efficacy of treatment. It may also be of use to identify their beliefs about the motives of their physicians or treatment teams, as this may affect their perceptions of the probable impact of the recommended treatment.

Suggested Questions

- "Tell me what you really believe is wrong with your health now."
- "Do you believe that you need some kind of treatment?"
- "What is treatment likely to do for you? Why do you think it will have that effect?"
- "What do you believe will happen if you are not treated?"
- "Why do you think your doctor has recommended [specific treatment] for you?"

As we noted in Chapter 3, patients may have many reasons for disagreeing with their physicians' conclusions about their conditions and the treatment that they need. Only when patients' beliefs are based on the effects of psychopathology, such as delusions, depressive hopelessness, or the denial frequently seen in manic states, is their failure to appreciate the nature of their situation and its consequences of relevance to their competence. Therefore, when patients' views of their situation do not comport with the perspectives of their physicians, it is crucial to ascertain the reasons for the beliefs that they hold. Similarly, when patients' stated preferences are at odds with previous decisions they have made, clinicians should be alerted to the need to explore what is behind these inconsistencies.

When it is unclear whether realistic or delusional reasoning underlies a patient's view, it may be helpful to pose a hypothetical question that challenges the basis for the patient's belief to see whether his or her reasoning is flexible enough to adapt to new input. For example, patients who deny that any medication may be helpful could be asked whether they would feel the same way about a new medication they had never tried that had been found to help 90% of people with problems just like theirs. If patients' denial is based on the delusion that no medication will help them because they are being punished by God for their sins, they are likely to refuse to acknowledge any possibility of a positive effect. Other patients, however, who doubt the efficacy of medication only because of previous experiences with ineffective treatments, should be more capable of acknowledging some chance of benefit in the hypothetical situation being described.

Ability to reason with relevant information. The essence of this standard is whether patients can use the information they have been given to engage in a process of weighing treatment options. Because no one achieves the ideal of a rational decision maker (of which Spock and Data in the *Star Trek* television and movie series are the fictional exemplars), patients are not expected to weigh risks and benefits in a computerlike fashion. Emotional factors, which patients may have difficulty putting into words, should and will inevitably enter into their deliberations (DiMasio, 1995). Rather, we are looking for evidence that patients have taken the major factors into account, considered the options, and reached a conclusion roughly congruent with their starting premises. Moreover, as with Appreciation, we are particularly concerned with impairments of Reasoning based on mental or cognitive disorders.

Suggested Questions

- "Tell me how you reached the decision to accept [reject] the recommended treatment."

- "What were the factors that were important to you in reaching the decision?"
- "How did you balance those factors?"

The questions suggested here are only examples of how patients might be queried about their decision-making abilities. As examiners gain experience, they may want to develop their own sets of questions that embody their particular styles of interacting with patients. Most important, however, is to have a structure for the assessment, so that all the data about the patient's capacities that can be obtained from a direct examination are in hand at the end of the interview.

Evaluating the Patient's General Mental Status

Even though the determinants of whether patients are competent to make treatment decisions are their decisional abilities *per se*, assessments should include a psychiatric history and a general mental status examination. Such examinations usually include consideration of patients' appearance, behavior, psychomotor performance, mood and affect, thought content and form, insight, judgment, and intellectual functioning. This overview of mental state should help the evaluator to determine whether impairments in performance are due to mental disorders or to other factors (e.g., the patient's disinclination to cooperate with the assessment), which may be directly relevant to the conclusion that is reached about the patient's decision-making capacities. Moreover, if a mental disorder is identified, the examiner will be in a position to suggest treatment interventions that might restore the patient's ability to make decisions.

Obtaining a psychiatric history and performing the mental status examination *after* the more focused evaluation of decision-making capacities is probably desirable for at least two reasons. First, much information relevant to the mental status examination is likely to be gathered by the examiner in the course of assessing the patient's decisional capacities, sparing the necessity of asking additional questions. In addition, given that some patients will have limited energy or attention spans, or will not tolerate the formal tasks involved in mental status assessment, there is a clear advantage in addressing decisional abilities while the patient is still fresh and cooperative.

How useful are psychological or neuropsychological tests in evaluating mental state in cases of suspected incompetence? In most cases, a clinical interview and mental status evaluation will provide all the information necessary for the decision. Some situations in which the nature or presence of a mental disorder is in question may benefit from psychological testing. In particular, selected neuropsychological tests can be of assistance, especially when frontal lobe impairment is suspected of affecting the patient's reasoning ability (Freedman, Stuss, & Gordon, 1991). And, at least for persons with Alzheimer's disease, a simple screening instrument aimed at detecting organic impairment, like the Mini-Mental State Examination, can be helpful in identifying patients who may require more careful evaluation.

Using Adjunctive Sources of Information

In contrast to the typical medical evaluation of a competent adult, assessments of decision-making capacity may require obtaining information from sources other than the patient. Family members and friends may be able to describe changes in the patient's level of functioning that are simply not apparent in a single examination. They may also be aware of deficits that the patient has successfully covered over during interactions with the evaluator. Some patients, for example, will have sufficient awareness to know that if they discuss their delusions openly, they may lose the power to make decisions for themselves. Only people who are present at less guarded moments will be able to report on the presence of these clinical phenomena.

Other caregivers can also provide critical information. Nursing staff members on an inpatient unit have an opportunity to observe patients over a period of time, and to judge the consistency of their behavior and their interactions with other people. Primary care physicians and treating mental health professionals in the community may also have invaluable information related to the patient's history and mental state. Medical and psychiatric records can help an evaluator assess whether a finding represents the patient's baseline state, or is indicative of a mental disorder of recent onset that may be adversely impacting their ability to make a choice.

Whenever possible, information should be sought from these adjunctive sources. It is well to keep in mind, however, that third parties often have their own interests in portraying patients as more or less capable than they really are. Family members, for instance, may want to override the patient's decision to refuse life-sustaining treatment, or to use the patient's putative incompetence to make treatment decisions as a launching pad for an effort to have the patient declared globally incompetent. Thus, evaluators should be alert to the possibility of bias in third-party reports and, when feasible, attempt to confirm their accounts from more objective sources.

TECHNIQUES TO MAXIMIZE PATIENTS' PERFORMANCE

When patients manifest serious deficits in their abilities to make treatment decisions, there are good reasons why an attempt to correct or compensate for those deficits should be considered an essential part of the evaluation. From a principled perspective, given the importance of the value of autonomy, it is always desirable to aid patients in retaining the right to make their own decisions. From a practical point of view, the likelihood of a successful treatment outcome often is enhanced by maintaining the patient's motivation and commitment to treatment, which is more likely if the patient is involved in making the treatment decision.

A key element in attempting to maximize patients' performance is delaying the final decision about their capacities. Except in emergencies, it is preferable not to rush into a judgment that the patient is incompetent. A repeat evaluation hours or days later is often helpful in distinguishing between time-limited and permanent impairments. For example, an injured patient brought to an emergency room following a car accident in which a loved one was killed may have a difficult time making a coherent decision. Things may be very different the following morning, as the patient achieves a measure of emotional stability. The same may be true for patients who have just learned that they have a life-threatening illness. In cases like these, when there is reason to believe that patients' normally adequate abilities to grasp and process information are impaired by stress, allowing them to delay the decision for a short period of time — in some cases just a few hours — may give them a chance to adapt to the initial trauma of their circumstances before making a treatment decision.

Even when some degree of decisional impairment is likely to persist, delay in passing judgment and initiating treatment offers the opportunity to address those factors that may deprive the patient of decision-making power. To conceptualize this, recall our observation in Chapter 2 that "competence" or "incompetence" is a conclusion about the "match or mismatch between [the person's] abilities and the decision-making demands of the situation that the person faces."

Appropriate interventions, therefore, may involve modifying the procedures for obtaining consent to compensate for patients' impairments, identifying the underlying causes of patients' decisional difficulties and acting to ameliorate them, or both.

> In Chapter 3, we described a 69-year-old woman with severe vasoconstriction of a finger who was approached by her surgeon to discuss destruction of nerve tissue in her stellate ganglion, with the aim of relaxing the constricted blood vessels. The patient initially agreed to have the procedure, but as the surgeon discussed the risks and benefits, she said that she did not want to hear about them and withdrew her consent. A psychiatric consultant, after a similar experience with the patient, concluded that her anxiety level was so high that it was interfering with her ability to attend to the disclosure. She recommended small doses of an antianxiety agent, and that the treatment team call in the patient's neighbor, her main social contact, to be with the patient as the disclosure took place. Instead, on the assumption that if the patient were now unable to tolerate disclosure then she was permanently incompetent, her attending physician discharged her from the hospital without further treatment.

The attending surgeon's misconception that a decision about the patient's competence had to be made immediately, and that it was illegitimate to take steps to improve her decision making, led to this patient failing to receive the care that she clearly needed. Had the surgeon accepted the consultant's reasonable recommendations for attempting to improve the patient's ability to listen to the disclosure (or been knowledgeable about the patient's right to waive disclosure), there is a good chance that the patient would have been able to consent to care.

The options we review here for maximizing patients' decision-making abilities are not exhaustive. Creativity, informed by the clinician's understanding of a specific patient, will often lead to the identification of new techniques for assisting patients to make meaningful decisions.

Enhancing Disclosure of Information

Some patients who fail to grasp the information relevant to a treatment decision can be helped to attain adequate understanding by modification of disclosure techniques and some "teaching" on the part of the evaluator. The following are among the approaches that can be tried.

Written disclosures. Patients may grasp disclosures better if they are given a written version to study after a verbal explanation. Part of the benefit may derive from having some time alone to reflect while reviewing the information. In addition, some people simply acquire and process information better when they read it, rather than merely hearing it. Of course, the value of this approach is tied closely to the readability of the written disclosure, which involves elimination of technical terms and medical jargon, as well as to the logical sequencing of the information. The MacCAT-T's progression of disclosure — disorder, recommended treatment, benefits/risks, alternative treatments — is one useful way to organize information (see Chapter 6). Treatment procedures themselves often are best understood when presented chronologically: from preparation for the intervention, to the procedure itself, to immediate and longer-term follow-up.

One might consider presenting some types of information twice in order to enhance the patient's ability both to understand and to reason about the data. For example, most disclosures will describe the recommended treatment at one point and the alternative treatments at another. It may often be worthwhile to have a summary that promotes meaningful comparison of the treatments. If Treatment A and Treatment B have different probabilities of success, the summary can state these in juxtaposition, rather than relying on the patient to "connect" the two pieces of information.

Teaching aids. Diagrams, illustrations, and models may be useful as patient education tools. Risks and benefits of alternative forms of treatment, for example, can be presented in tabular form so patients can make comparisons across treatment options. Illustrations and plastic models may help patients grasp the nature of physical traumas, organic dysfunctions, and proposed procedures. Videotapes are now increasingly available to assist with this task.

Translators. If English is not the patient's primary language — even if the patient can communicate in English — the clinician might consider whether a translator's assistance during the disclosure would be helpful. The translator might need to help only during those parts of the disclosure for which the patient is manifesting poor understanding. It can also be helpful to have the translator query the patient's understanding in his or her native tongue and convey the patient's explanation to the evaluator.

Addressing Psychodynamic Issues

Denial of the reality of illness or delusional explanations for medical problems (which generally impair patients' appreciation of their disorder or the possibilities for treatment) can be understood as patients' dysfunctional mechanisms for coping with stress. Sometimes the underlying anxieties to which these misperceptions are a response can be addressed successfully through short-term psychotherapeutic interventions.

A 74-year-old retired secretary with a history of paranoid psychosis was found to have a large lump in her breast. After biopsy and probable mastectomy were recommended, the administrator of the nursing home in which she lived requested an evaluation of her competence. When evaluated, the patient revealed a delusional belief that the surgeon who had diagnosed her later called to say that she really didn't need the surgery and that he had only recommended it because his wife needed more money. Careful exploration of her feelings about the procedure revealed a fear that, if she required mastectomy, she would then be a defective woman who would be abandoned by all of her caretakers and allowed to die. The evaluator empathized with these concerns and brought in the patient's continuing care nurse — an important person in her life — to underscore her commitment to the patient. As the patient recognized that surgery would not mean she was devalued as a person, her anxieties were alleviated, her delusions disappeared, and she consented to surgery, which was performed uneventfully.

Fears about death, deformity, and abandonment are common among patients with severe medical illnesses. Resulting psychotic defenses are often lowered as efforts are made to address these concerns. Sometimes, however, clinicians will use other techniques, such as direct confrontation of the distorted or delusional belief. They may also employ paradoxical approaches, such as expressing their agreement with the delusion. The latter may weaken the potency of the belief, as patients protest the absurdity of the view now endorsed by the evaluator. Whatever the approach taken, however, the key is to keep in mind the potential effect of psychodynamic factors on patients' mental states.

Pursuing Pharmacologic Interventions

Medications are a double-edged sword: they may contribute to patients' impaired decision making or may help to correct the problem. With many elderly and hospitalized patients taking multiple medications, one should always consider the possibility that the impairments detected are due to a pharmacologic effect. Analgesics and hypnotics are notorious for interfering with mentation, especially in the elderly. Antihypertensives, steroids, and cardiac medications, among others, can have similar effects. It is often worth seeing whether short-term discontinuation of suspect medications, as long as the patient's medical state permits, can alleviate the impairment in decisional capacity.

On the other hand, initiation of medication may sometimes be required. Analgesics may relieve pain that interferes with the patient's ability to attend to and process information. Medications that provide relief from psychosis, depression, or anxiety can have similar benefits. When endocrinologic or metabolic abnormalities underlie the disturbances in patients' mentation, correction of the problem often leaves patients in a position to make subsequent treatment decisions. If possible, decisions about definitive treatment should be delayed long enough to see whether changes in medication regimens are sufficient to restore decisional capacity.

Can patients whose competence is in question consent to these alterations in their treatment? In many cases, they can. As we noted in Chapter 2, the judgment that a patient may be incompetent to decide about one type of treatment does not necessarily mean that the patient is unable to make all decisions. Less capacity is required when a decision has few adverse consequences (e.g., a trial of an antidepressant) than when major risks are involved (e.g., abdominal surgery to remove a tumor). Thus, a clinician may accept a patient's consent for a change in medications even while questioning the patient's capacity to consent to other treatment.

Providing Situational Supports

Patients' difficulties in the consent process can sometimes be ameliorated by altering the social context to provide them with additional support. The presence of family members, friends, a trusted personal physician, a member of the clergy of the patient's faith, or even just a staff member of the same ethnic group can reduce the level of anxiety that patients feel in unfamiliar and threatening medical environments. Moreover, such persons can help patients process the information they have been given, often by reinterpreting it for them in language with which they are familiar and by clarifying distortions. Patients may also feel freer to reveal their confusion and to ask relevant questions in interactions with relatives and friends.

In some instances, patients will engage in a process of shared decision making with other persons, with both parties agreeing to a choice that neither could have reached alone. Patients may even choose to defer the judgment to a relative or friend, stating their willingness to accept whatever he or she decides. As long as patients understand the implications of handing effective decisional authority to a third party, they may be capable of making that choice, even if not able to make the ultimate decision about treatment on their own. When family members or friends are drawn into these roles, however, the clinician should ensure that they are adequately informed about the medical situation and treatment options. The clinician also needs to keep in mind that sometimes the cognitive or emotional limitations of these third parties or their conflicts of interest with the patient make them inappropriate choices for assisting the patient with a decision. (See Chapter 8 for a more detailed discussion of these issues.)

In addition to introducing familiar faces, other situational interventions may also be helpful. If patients have developed a conflictual relationship with a physician, such that they are unable or unwilling to collaborate with that person in making a treatment decision, it makes little sense to insist that such interactions continue. Responsibility for the patient's care should be transferred to someone with whom the patient can interact comfortably. As unfortunate as ethnic, religious, and racial prejudices are, when they interfere with doctor–patient communication, involving a new physician is often the simplest way to resolve the problem.

Finally, there are some commonsense means of adjusting the situation to facilitate decision making. Disclosure and discussions should take place in quiet surroundings so that distractions are minimized. Patients and relatives may also benefit from having a private place to which they can retreat to process information and make a decision. Medical settings are not always conducive to quiet reflection, but that opportunity is sometimes precisely what patients need.

SUMMARY

The assessment of patients' decision-making capacities can be performed by either the treating clinician or a consultant. Whoever performs the evaluation should be aware of the legal and ethical basis for the rules governing decision-making competence, and be knowledgeable about mental status evaluation.

At the outset of an assessment, a consultant should ascertain why the evaluation is being requested, which may provide important clues about the basis for the patient's suspected impairment. Patients should be informed about the purpose of the evaluation and given the information they would need to make a treatment decision, preferably by their attending physician or another member of the treatment team.

Evaluations should be structured according to the decision-making abilities relevant to the determination of competence in a particular jurisdiction. A set of standard questions can be helpful in insuring that key aspects of patients' functioning are not overlooked. After patients' functional abilities are explored, a formal mental status examination should be performed. This will help to determine the degree to which psychopathological factors are affecting patients' decision making. Information from third parties can also be important in assessing patients' functioning.

Because deprivation of decision-making power should be avoided whenever possible, evaluators ought to maximize patients' performance. This may require delaying a final decision about patients' competence while ameliorative interventions are attempted. Along these lines, disclosure of consent-related information can be enhanced, psychodynamic issues addressed, pharmacologic treatment attempted, and situational supports provided.

The clinical techniques discussed in this chapter can help attending physicians and consultants alike get the information they need to assess whether patients are capable of making their own decisions. In Chapter 6 we examine a more structured approach to assessment of decision-making capacities.

6

USING THE MacARTHUR COMPETENCE ASSESSMENT TOOL—TREATMENT

An important part of the process of assessing patients' capacities to make treatment decisions is the direct observation of their abilities to grasp the meaning of information provided (Understanding), recognize its relevance for themselves (Appreciation), use the information in a decision-making process (Reasoning), and offer a choice (Express a Choice). Now we describe a method that we have developed to assist clinicians in making these observations. The method is a structured interview and rating procedure called the "MacArthur Competence Assessment Tool for Treatment (the "MacCAT-T").

The Appendix provides the manual for the MacCAT-T, including basic instructions for its administration, a form to assist clinicians in organizing the interview and recording patients' responses, and a guide for rating responses. This chapter describes in more detail how to use the MacCAT-T. The instrument itself should be consulted as one proceeds through the chapter. The focus in this chapter is on getting the right kind of data and comparing it to MacCAT-T norms. Combining MacCAT-T results with other clinical data to arrive at judgments about competence will be described in Chapter 7. Readers who do not anticipate using an instrument like the MacCAT-T to aid in competence evaluations can proceed directly to Chapter 7, or they can read the first two following sections, which provide a brief overview of the instrument. Readers who want more detail about the instrument's development can consult Grisso, Appelbaum, and Hill-Fotouhi (in press). Bound copies of the manual, $8\frac{1}{2} \times 11$ record forms, and a training videotape for MacCAT-T administration are available from the authors.

OVERVIEW OF THE MacCAT-T

We developed the MacCAT-T to meet clinicians' need for a practical tool that would help them obtain and organize information about patients' decision-making abilities. For our previous research on patients' capacities to make treatment decisions (Appelbaum & Grisso, 1995; Grisso & Appelbaum, 1995 a, b; Grisso, Appelbaum, Mulvey, & Fletcher, 1995), we had developed several research instruments to assess patients' four abilities related to legal competence described in Chapter 3. Demands for scientific reliability resulted in instruments that were lengthy, involved rigorous and complex scoring criteria, and required standardization of procedures that did not allow information to be tailored to the specific circumstances of each patient. These instruments served the purposes of our research quite well, but have several limitations for ordinary clinical practice. The MacCAT-T, therefore, was developed in response to the need for a clinically usable instrument.

Our previous research suggested that the MacCAT-T should assess all four types of abilities associated with legal and ethical standards for patients' decision-making competence. How well patients performed in any one of these areas tended not to be a very good indicator of their performance on the other abilities. Not all of the four abilities might be relevant in all legal jurisdictions or clinical situations; but all would be relevant in some jurisdictions. Therefore, all were included as assessment objectives for the MacCAT-T.

We wanted the MacCAT-T to provide a way to assess these abilities within the context of a clinician–patient dialogue, patterned on a procedure for obtaining informed consent for treatment. The method had to be short enough that it would not tax patients' often limited capacities for attention and would be responsive to limits on clinicians' time. Moreover, the procedure had to allow clinicians to assess patients' abilities with reference to patients' own specific disorders, treatment options, and life circumstances rather than to hypothetical situations. Thus the format needed to be sufficiently flexible for use in assessing patients with a wide range of illnesses, including psychiatric disorders.

The MacCAT-T, therefore, is a structured interview, usually requiring about 15 to 20 minutes to complete, that follows a fixed sequence of topics. The MacCAT-T guides the clinician through a disclosure of patients' own disorders and treatment options. The disclosure, however, is not a mechanical and one-sided communication *to* the patient. It is interspersed with questions that require feedback *from* the patient. This feedback is used to assess the degree to which patients are Understanding the information and recognizing (Appreciating) the relevance of the information for their own situation. The MacCAT-T then guides the clinician to explore how patients are thinking through the treatment decision so as to arrive at a picture of their Reasoning abilities.

The MacCAT-T comes with a record form that

- allows the clinician to organize the specific content of his or her informed consent disclosure prior to meeting with the patient;
- provides the clinician a visual guide for conducting the interview while talking to the patient;
- allows the clinician to keep organized notes describing the patient's responses to the various inquiries that contribute to the assessment of the patient's decision-making abilities;
- facilitates the clinician's rating procedure after the interview is completed; and
- acts as documentation of the dialogue, providing a record to which the clinician may refer when asked to describe data and logic for the clinician's judgment about the patient's capacities in later clinical consultations or legal inquiries.

The nature of the MacCAT-T, of course, does preclude its use with certain patients who are nonverbal: for example, some persons with profound mental retardation, patients on respirators, patients in mute catatonic states, and individuals manifesting severe delirium.

Because of the value of quantitative descriptions of patients' abilities, the MacCAT-T provides a system for rating their responses. Assigning ratings helps to identify points of agreement between clinicians, as well as points of disagreement that are in need of clarification. Quantitative ways to express patients' degrees of ability also allow for the development of norms to which clinicians can compare individual cases. This assists clinicians in making comparative statements about patients' capacities, such as expressing a patient's degree of deficit in relation to the capacities of other patients or nonpatients.

In developing the rating system, we opted for an approach that allows a fair amount of clinical discretion. The rating system offers clinicians broad concepts with which to "anchor" their ratings, while not being tied to highly detailed scoring rules. The alternative would have been to develop rather complex scoring criteria — like those used in our research measures — that may have discouraged some clinicians from adopting the MacCAT-T for routine use. Moreover, the MacCAT-T's use of content that is tailored to the patient's own unique circumstances discouraged the development of very rigid and specific scoring criteria. The result, therefore, is a system that anchors clinicians' ratings to broad concepts while allowing flexibility and discretion. Whatever has been sacrificed by way of potential psychometric precision is for the sake of greater practical utility.

There is an inherent danger in an assessment system that assigns ratings or scores to patients' decision-making abilities. Clinicians or the persons to whom they communicate the results may be tempted to presume that the assessment system has measured competence itself, and that legal or ethical questions about competence can be answered on the basis of the patient's numerical rating.

Practice based on this presumption, however, would constitute a misuse of MacCAT-T ratings. There is a great difference between measuring the level of patients' decision-making capacities (the objective of the MacCAT-T) and deciding whether they will be allowed to make autonomous choices (the objective of clinical or legal decisions about competence). The former may assist with the latter, but no particular level of capacity can stand for competence or incompetence across cases.

OVERVIEW OF ADMINISTRATION AND RATING

The MacCAT-T interview is a relatively simple procedure that requires only a few minutes of preparation, about 20 minutes for the interview itself, and 2 or 3 minutes for rating responses. Here we describe the various parts of the process. Remaining sections of the chapter discuss each of these same steps at a greater level of detail, which might be of interest to clinicians who use the MacCAT-T in research, as a training tool, or as a method in cases that are likely to be scrutinized by courts.

To prepare for the MacCAT-T interview, the clinician develops a brief description of the patient's disorder, the recommended treatment, and the treatment's benefits and risks/discomforts. For each of these topics, the clinician writes in the spaces provided on the Mac-CAT-T Record Form each of the pieces of information to be disclosed to the patient. (See the copy of the MacCAT-T Record Form in the Appendix.) Aspects of the disorder are recorded on page 1, the last space being a description of the probable course of the disorder if no treatment were to be received. Important information regarding the nature of the recommended treatment is written in on page 2, and at least two benefits and two risks/discomforts of the treatment are recorded on page 3. A separate one-page form, called the Alternative Treatment Form, has similar spaces for preparing disclosures of each alternative treatment.

The steps in the procedure are described in the paragraphs that follow:

Understanding of Disorder

The MacCAT-T interview begins with the clinician disclosing to the patient the prepared description of the disorder. After this description, the clinician asks the patient to describe, "in your own words," what the clinician has disclosed about the disorder. The clinician records the patient's responses in the spaces provided on page 1 of the Record Form. If the patient appears to have difficulty with any of the information, the clinician attempts to "teach" the patient about it and reassesses the patient's grasp of the information.

Appreciation of Disorder

Before disclosing further information, the clinician assesses the patient's appreciation of the relevance of the description of disorder for his or her own condition (". . . do you believe that you have these symptoms?"). Whatever the patient's responses, the clinician engages the patient in a brief discussion of the reasons for his or her belief and records the patient's explanation.

Understanding of Treatment and Risks/Discomforts

The next two sections (pages 2 and 3 of the Record Form) involve disclosure of the recommended treatment and its benefits and risks, eliciting the patient's demonstration of Understanding, and recording the patient's responses, in a process similar to the Understanding of Disorder section.

Appreciation of Treatment

Here patients are asked whether it is possible that the treatment might be of some benefit to them. Whether the patient says "yes" or "no" is not important at this point. What is being assessed are patients' explanations for their beliefs about treatment, especially whether they involve clearly false, distorted, or delusional ideas pertaining to the treatment.

Alternative Treatments

The clinician now discloses treatments and benefits/risks for each of the relevant alternative treatments. This procedure of disclosure and questions concerning the patient's understanding is identical to the one used earlier for the recommended treatment.

Reasoning

The patient is next asked to make a treatment choice. Once the preference is stated, the patient is asked to explain what makes it seem
better than the alternatives. The patient's explanation, which the clinician records on page 4 of the Record Form, will be rated later for the
patient's ability to think about options in terms of their consequences,
and to make comparisons between options.

A second Reasoning procedure (page 5 of Record Form) asks patients to imagine any "everyday" consequences of their preferred treatment, then of the treatment they do not prefer. The objective here is
to determine if the patient is capable of going beyond the purely
"medical" benefits and risks that have been disclosed (e.g., "The medication may make you dizzy"), to make inferences about how they
would influence the patient's everyday functioning in practical activities (e.g., "I might not be able to operate the lathe at work").

Expressing a Choice

Finally, the patient is asked to state a treatment choice in light of
everything that has now been considered.

Rating Patient Responses

The MacCAT-T Manual (see Appendix) provides simple criteria for
rating the adequacy of patients' responses on each item of the various
sections of the MacCAT-T interview. The clinician records the ratings
in the spaces by each item on pages 1 to 5, and on page 6 they are
summarized to produce ratings for Understanding, Appreciation, Reasoning, and Expressing a Choice.

Although the MacCAT-T interview has many sections and topics, it
is not as daunting to administer as it might seem from this discussion.
Clinicians whom we have trained in the MacCAT-T procedure have
felt comfortable with it after only two or three interviews. This is probably because the Record Form acts as a reminder of the sequence of
topics and provides prompts for the clinician. Moreover, the "flow" of

the procedure follows a logical sequence of topics that feels natural to most clinicians.

The remaining sections of the chapter describe in more detail the steps we have just reviewed. They discuss issues of administration that have been raised primarily in our training of psychiatric residents and in research situations where careful attention to standardization has been desirable.

PREPARING FOR THE MacCAT-T INTERVIEW

To prepare for the MacCAT-T interview, the clinician selects the information that will be disclosed and notes that information on the Record Form (Fig. A.1). The specific information that clinicians choose will vary in relation to two possible purposes for clinicians' use of the MacCAT-T. In some cases, clinicians will be interested primarily in getting a sample of the patients' functioning on the four abilities: Understanding, Appreciation, Reasoning, and Expressing a Choice. This purpose can be fulfilled without disclosing everything that might be relevant for patients' treatment decisions. Disclosure can be built around information that is typical of what must be understood without necessarily covering all of the things that patients might need to know.

In other cases, clinicians might want to use the MacCAT-T to provide not only an assessment, but also a documentation of patients' Understanding, Appreciation and Reasoning concerning all of the information and alternative treatments that are relevant for their situations. This might be desirable in some complex cases that require judicial review. When used for this purpose, the information disclosed in the MacCAT-T procedure must be more comprehensive.

For convenience, the following discussions will refer to these two purposes as the "assessment" objective (getting a sample of the patient's abilities) and the "documentation" objective (covering the full range of things that the patient must know).

Preparing for Disclosure of the Disorder   record form p. 1

Preparing to disclose the disorder to the patient requires three things: (1) a knowledge of the patient's disorder, (2) the selection of two or three primary features of the disorder, and (3) a general knowledge of what is likely to happen if the disorder progresses (without treatment). Let us examine these in turn.

Type of disorder   space 1, p. 1

The clinician enters the name of the disorder that requires treatment. Judgments about whether to use simplified terms (e.g., "a cancer of the stomach") or technical terms (e.g., "a mental disorder called Cyclothymic Disorder") are at the discretion of the clinician. If technical terms are used, however, they should be followed by a simplified, descriptive phrase (e.g., "That's a mood disorder in which you swing back and forth between being somewhat excited and somewhat depressed").

Description of disorder   spaces 2–4, p. 1

The clinician makes at least two, but preferably three, entries that describe the nature of the disorder and/or its symptoms. This number is required for evaluations that are fulfilling only assessment objectives; evaluations that also have documentation objectives will require listing as many aspects of the disorder as are considered relevant for meeting informed consent requirements for adequate disclosure.

Ways to describe disorders may include references to a disease process, sequelae of the disease, and/or symptoms that patients typically experience with the disorder. Which of these are chosen for the disclosure may vary with the type of disorder. For example, a disclosure for deep venous thrombosis is likely to include a description of physical aspects of the disorder focusing on blood vessels, clots, and the process of their migration, whereas a disclosure for schizophrenia is unlikely to include (but might) a description of chemical abnormalities in neurotransmitters. Descriptions associated with mental disorders are more likely to focus on cognitive, affective, and behavioral symptoms of the disorder (e.g., "hallucinations: seeing things that other people do not believe are there").

Untreated course of the disorder   space 5, p. 1
  Here the clinician enters a description of the probable outcome of the disease process if it were allowed to run its course without treatment. For example, in the context of life-threatening diseases, the entry may be a brief description of the likely outcome (e.g., "Few people left untreated survive more than a year"). For mental disorders, the entry may refer to likely persistence of the disorder's cognitive or affective symptoms, with concomitant functional disability.

Preparing for Disclosure of the Treatment   record form p. 2

Preparing to disclose a treatment to the patient requires a decision about the treatment that will be recommended, and the selection of two or three things that patients should know about how the treatment is carried out.

Type of treatment   space 1, p. 2
  The clinician enters the name of the treatment that is being recommended, or a phrase that identifies the treatment intervention. The purpose of this entry is to label the treatment for the patient, whether it be a surgical procedure or a psychopharmacological intervention. With psychoactive medication, the name of the medication should be identified.

Description of treatment   spaces 2–4, p. 2
  The purpose here is to tell factually what is involved in performing the treatment or accomplishing the intervention (not its benefits or risks). For example, a description of the use of a psychoactive medication might refer to the route by which the medication is administered (e.g., oral or intravenous), how often and when it is administered, conditions under which it should not be administered (e.g., in combination with other medications), how long one may have to take the medication before its therapeutic effect is likely to be apparent, or whether continued use of the medication is necessary in order to

maintain its therapeutic effect. For surgical procedures, entries might include references to anesthesia, a brief summary of the surgical task, and some aspects of postoperative care such as necessary rehabilitative activities.

The events and procedures that need to be described will often be more lengthy when the MacCAT-T is being used not only for assessment but also for documentation of the informed consent process. Points of description beyond the three that are needed for assessment purposes can be listed in the "Other" space at the bottom of p. 2 of the Record Form. Entries in spaces 2–4 may be those that are considered to have somewhat greater importance as features that the patient should understand.

Preparing for Disclosure of the Benefits/Risks   *record form, p. 3*

Here the objective is to describe to the patient a few expected benefits of the treatment, as well as a few potential risks or discomforts of the treatment. When uses of the MacCAT-T are limited to assessment objectives, only two benefits (spaces 1 and 2, p. 3) and two risks (spaces 3 and 4, p. 3) are needed. For purposes of documenting a full informed consent procedure, one may use the "Other" entry space at the bottom of p. 3.

Describing benefits and risks. Benefits will usually refer to such things as reduction in symptoms (e.g., "hallucinations will go away"), physical gains (e.g., "You will gain mobility—You can walk around unaided"), or extension of life (e.g., "will reduce the risk of future heart attacks").

"Risks" is a shorthand term to refer to any important consequences of the treatment that may be undesirable. Some of these may be aspects of the treatment that place the patient in some jeopardy (e.g., tardive dyskinesia as a consequence of neuroleptic medication, adverse reactions to anesthesia). Other possible entries, however, include discomforts (e.g., "You might have brief periods of dizziness") or limitations (e.g., "This approach will only give you 50% extension of your knee," or "The plastic hip joint could wear out in time and have to be replaced").

Describing "chances." The MacCAT-T rating system requires that each Benefit and Risk entry include a statement of its chances of happening — the likelihood of the benefit or risk for the patient in question. For example, a patient may be told that "most people experience dizziness," or "the likelihood that you will experience pain in your leg after the surgical incisions have healed is very low." These statements of likelihood will be offered to the patient when each benefit or risk is disclosed, and patients will be rated in part on their understanding of these likelihoods.

We recommend that chances or likelihoods be stated in quite general terms, unless there is compelling reason to state them more specifically. By general terms, we mean broad phrases such as "most people," "usually," "only in rare cases," "almost always," or "sometimes." Although such terms lack precision, the alternatives also have their limitations. For example, offering a specific percentage probability often conveys greater certainty about the chances than our medical knowledge can support. Moreover, if odds are being adjusted in response to some specific characteristic of the patient that places him or her on the low or high side compared to the norm, stating the odds numerically often is no more precise than using verbal shorthand to offer a general sense of the chances.

Nevertheless, some clinicians may feel that there are times when it is important to express the chances of benefits or risks numerically, rather than relying on more general phrases. When this is the case, we recommend that the chances be described as frequencies rather than percents. For example, rather than disclosing that there is a "20 percent chance" of a particular side-effect, inform the patient that "2 out of 10 people" who take the medication experience the side-effect. Odds expressed as percents require somewhat more ability to think abstractly than do statements of numerical frequency.

Preparing for Disclosure of Alternative Treatments

The Alternative Treatment (AT) Form (Fig. A.2) is identical in format to the sections of the MacCAT-T form just described for planning disclosure of the recommended treatment. The AT Form is used in two ways depending on the clinician's objectives.

First, if the MacCAT-T is being used in a case in order to provide both assessment and documentation of a complete informed consent process, that will require disclosure of all relevant alternatives to the recommended treatment. In these cases, the clinician should prepare an AT Form for each of the alternative treatments to be disclosed. The manner of preparing the AT Form is identical to that for the disclosure of the recommended treatment.

Second, if the MacCAT-T is being used in a case in which the objective is only to assess the patient's decision-making abilities, then the clinician will need to decide on only one alternative treatment to disclose and will complete only one AT Form. This disclosure is necessary because a later part of the MacCAT-T process (pertaining to Reasoning abilities) requires that the patient compare the recommended treatment to an alternative. Patients' understanding of the disclosure of the alternative treatment does not need to be rated. Therefore, when completing the AT Form in this type of case, the clinician may shorten the disclosure by preparing only two statements describing the treatment, and only one benefit and one risk.

General Guidelines for Obtaining and Formatting Relevant Information for the Disclosure

Preparation involved in all of the steps noted — for disclosing the disorder, the recommended treatment, its benefits/risks, and alternative treatment — requires that clinicians obtain information and format it properly. A careful review of the most recent clinical information in the patient's medical chart is a requirement, at a minimum, for obtaining this information.

Most highly recommended, however, is a consultation with the patient's treating clinician. This has benefits in addition to maximizing the relevance of the disclosure for the patient's situation. It can be used to enlist the treating clinician's collaboration in the informed consent process, which may enhance ongoing communications between doctor and patient. It also guards against the possibility that the patient will receive contradictory information from the treating clinician and the assessing clinician.

Clinicians will encounter two uncertainties in the process of preparing their descriptions of disorders for disclosure to patients: How much do patients need to know? And how should the descriptions be worded?

When the MacCAT-T is used for the assessment objective alone (i.e., documentation of the full informed consent process is not the purpose), patients do not need to be told all of the details that might be relevant for an actual treatment decision. A very basic, often over-simplified description will be sufficient, as long as it touches on the main points of the disorder.

When the MacCAT-T is being used for the documentation objective, however, the guidelines to be applied are those that we discussed in Chapter 5. The disorder must be described in as much detail as the average patient, or this specific patient, would want to have in order to make an informed choice. Generally this requires a more extensive and detailed description than we suggest when the MacCAT-T is used only to meet assessment objectives.

The rule of thumb for selecting wording is to use terms and language that maximize the likelihood of understanding by the patient. For the majority of adolescents and adults in the United States, this means a level of word difficulty and sentence length that is more like one finds in articles in small-town newspapers than in the *New Yorker*, and more akin to talking about one's work in a seventh- or eighth-grade classroom than in an undergraduate lecture hall.

PERFORMING THE MacCAT-T INTERVIEW

The MacCAT-T interview is standardized in three important ways. First, it provides a *fixed sequence* with which particular types of information are given and questions are asked. Second, in many parts of the MacCAT-T the questions themselves use *specific wording* that is intended for use with all patients. Third, *cues to probe* for additional information occur at various points in the MacCAT-T interview. When clinicians want to use the procedure in its most standardized fashion (e.g., for research, or for cases that may receive judicial scrutiny), they should adhere carefully to these features of the MacCAT-T.

Even when one uses the MacCAT-T in the most standardized way, the interview process should not be rigid or mechanical. In our own use of the MacCAT-T with many patients, medical and psychiatric, we have recognized a number of ways in which the MacCAT-T interview should flex in response to individual differences among patients.

One of these is the pace of the interview. The sensitive clinician will adjust to a patient's apparent need to go more slowly through the interview, or the patient's apparent ability to move right along. In addition, we find that, especially with psychiatric patients, one must tolerate patients' occasional divergence from the path of the interview, for example, as a consequence of the patient's loose associations, or the patient's need to express some distress regarding other events of the day. Clinical common sense and skill will allow one to recognize and respond to such events thoughtfully, while keeping them brief and guiding the patient back to the point of divergence from the interview.

With these general considerations in mind, let us review the specific parts of the MacCAT-T administration as they are outlined in the Record Form. More specific instructions for each of these parts are provided in the MacCAT-T manual in the Appendix. Page citations here refer to the Record Form.

Disclosure of Disorder

The material that the clinician has entered into the five spaces (p. 1) is used to fashion a description of the disorder. The clinician then says to the patient, "I want to make sure you understand this before we go on. Tell me in your own words what I've described about the disorder." Patients may be cued to provide specific types of information if they leave them out of their initial descriptions (e.g., "Do you recall what I called this disorder?"). If one of the elements seems to have been misunderstood, only partially understood, or not recalled, the clinician then presents it again and reinquires concerning the patient's understanding. However, if more than one element is "missed" in the first disclosure and inquiry process, it is best for the clinician to do a complete redisclosure of the information about the disorder before reinquiring.

When recording patients' responses, the clinician need not write down every word. Our practice is to write down the critical phrase(s) that the patient offers relating to the five elements in the disclosure. We try to do this as close to verbatim as possible, which greatly facilitates our explanations of patients' understanding in later clinical consultations or queries by courts.

Appreciation of Disorder

The purpose of this procedure (p. 2) is to determine whether patients believe that the information just provided to them actually applies to them, that is, whether they agree or disagree that they have the disorder and symptoms that have just been described. Nothing new is disclosed. The wording of the inquiry should be followed closely.

Probing often will be necessary. If the patient indicates disagreement with the description, the clinician explores the specific nature of the patient's disagreement. Is it disbelief about the diagnosis, all the symptoms, or only some of the symptoms? Then patients are asked to explain their disagreement with the description as it applies to themselves. Modest challenges may be offered (e.g., "Your doctor says that you were complaining of chest pains just yesterday"). These are not intended to modify the patient's belief, and they should not be worded as attempts to persuade. Their purpose is evaluative, to determine whether the patient rigidly holds the belief being expressed or whether it is held with ambivalence.

The critical parts of the response should be written in the space provided as close to verbatim as possible. The interview proceeds, however, even if the patient is in disagreement.

Disclosure of Treatment

This procedure (p. 2) is very like the one described above for Disclosure of Disorder.

Disclosure of Benefits/Risks

In this procedure (p. 3), which also is much like the one described for Disclosure of Disorder, all of the benefits and risks are disclosed before one makes the inquiry. The inquiry, however, may be made in two parts, first for the benefits and then for the risks.

Appreciation of Treatment

The purpose here (p. 4) is to determine whether patients believe that there might be *any* potential benefit from the treatment that has been described in the previous disclosure. Notice that the inquiry is worded in a way that tries to avoid asking the patient to make any commitments to the treatment. The objective is not to determine whether the patient will (or might) consent to this treatment. (Their agreement or disagreement with the value of the treatment will have no bearing on the rating that will be given for this section.) The purpose is to determine whether the patient has any delusional or bizarre beliefs about the potential value, or lack of potential value, of the treatment. Therefore, patients are asked – whether they agree or disagree with the treatment's value – to explain their evaluation of the treatment. That explanation is recorded by the clinician as faithfully as possible.

Alternative Treatments

As described earlier in the "Preparation" section, the clinician will have prepared one or more AT Forms describing alternative treatments. These are administered just like the Disclosure of Treatment and Disclosure of Benefits/Risks sections for the recommended treatment. When the MacCAT-T is being used only to obtain a sample of relevant abilities, the AT responses will not be rated. Therefore, less detailed attention may be given to the patient's understanding of the information, although the inquiry questions should still be asked.

First Choice and Reasoning

This section begins a process (p. 4) of exploring the patient's reasons for reaching a choice about treatment. After the recommended and alternative treatments are summarized, patients are invited to make an initial choice. They are then asked to describe how they arrived at the choice: ". . . what is it that makes that seem better than the others?" As the patient gives the explanation, the clinician explores it. Careful recording of patients' responses is important here, in order to be able to rate the "consequential" and "comparative" qualities of their reasoning.

Consequences

The purpose of this task (p. 5) is to examine the degree to which patients are able to go beyond the ordinary medical and psychiatric benefits/risks that have been described, to generate their own inferences about specific, practical differences that various outcomes might have in their lives. The emphasis, therefore, is on directing patients to consider the implications of their treatment choices for their everyday activities and the things that they especially value.

The procedure requires posing an inquiry question focused on the treatment for which the patient has expressed a preference ("First Choice," p. 4). Then the question is posed again for a treatment that the patient has rejected. The clinician may use any of the alternative treatments for this second question, or the recommended treatment if the patient has not chosen it. Then the patient is asked to explain how the benefits and discomforts of the treatment might "influence your everyday activities at home or work."

We have found that we must use probes quite liberally in this task. Patients often begin with answers that are very general (e.g., "I'll feel better — my life will be more comfortable"). Probes may simply take their cues from such comments and add the last stem from the original question (e.g., "How would 'feeling better' influence your everyday activities at home or at work?"). Credit has been achieved when patients state some relatively concrete consequence that is different from the immediate medical/psychiatric benefits or risks that were in the disclosure process (e.g., "If my emotions were better, I wouldn't yell at my kids so much"). We generally desist and move on, however, if patients have not provided such answers after about three probes of the type described above.

Final Choice

This procedure simply involves eliciting patients' final choices after having engaged in the process of explaining their original choice. Usually it has not changed, but sometimes the experience of explaining their choice has caused them to reconsider and to change their preferences. Nothing more is needed than to record the patient's final choice.

(The last part of p. 5 of the Record Form — "Logical Consistency of Choice" — is completed by the clinician during the rating process. It does not involve any separate task or inquiry while interviewing the patient.)

RATING THE RESPONSES

Complete instructions for rating individual responses are provided in a section ("III. Rating") of the MacCAT-T manual in the Appendix. Clinicians will find that there is considerable room for discretion in deciding whether patients' responses meet full (2 points), partial (1 point), or no (0) credit. In devising the rating guidelines, we struck a balance between highly specific criteria and very general criteria. The former would have provided greater precision, but the necessary detail and complexity would have been daunting and unwieldy for routine clinical uses of the MacCAT-T. Very general criteria, on the other hand, would have provided too little guidance for the rating process and would have risked a high degree of discrepancy between raters.

We suggest that when clinicians are uncertain about rating a patient's response in a higher or lower category, in general they should use the higher rating in order to avoid potentially "penalizing" patients unfairly. In addition, one will often find that patients give an inadequate answer, followed by an adequate answer to the same question after probing or some degree of reflection. In these instances, the general rule is to rate both the original and later responses, then record the rating for whichever response was better.

The present system, despite its flexibility, resulted in high degrees of interrater agreement in the MacCAT-T field studies. Interclass correlations for summary ratings between three raters, rating 40 cases (20 mentally ill and 20 non-ill), were .99 for Understanding, .87 for Appreciation, and .91 for Reasoning.

The MacCAT-T Rating Summary form (see Appendix) can be used to combine ratings to arrive at summary ratings for the four abilities assessed with the MacCAT-T.

The MacCAT-T does not yield a "Total" MacCAT-T rating because it would have little meaning empirically. The method is structured around four types of abilities, and our research suggests that patients may perform quite well on one ability while performing very poorly on another. In such cases, combining the ratings to suggest that the patient has overall "average" ability would ignore the fact that poor ability in any one area may be a critical deficit for purposes of judgments about competence. That the patient does very well in one ability does not necessarily compensate for a serious deficit in another ability.

Combining abilities to produce an overall MacCAT-T rating also would have limited meaning in light of differences among legal jurisdictions in standards for competence. Some states, for example, do not use a legal standard for competence that is conceptually related to the Reasoning component of the MacCAT-T. MacCAT-T ratings, therefore, are organized in a way that allows professionals to examine patients' performance on separate abilities and to take any of them into account to the extent that they are relevant from the legal or ethical perspective of the clinician or court that is using the results.

USING MacCAT-T RATINGS

The use of MacCAT-T ratings and other data for interpretations and judgments about patients' competence to make treatment decisions will be discussed in Chapter 7. To assist clinicians in this interpretative process, we performed field studies with the MacCAT-T to collect data with which clinicians can compare their patients' performance to that of subjects in our normative samples.

Our samples included 40 patients who were hospitalized with schizophrenia or schizoaffective disorder at the time they completed the MacCAT-T, and 40 individuals who were not mentally ill and who were residing in the community. These two groups were matched, person for person, on gender, age, race, and socioeconomic status (see Table 6.1). Most of the patients were interviewed within 6 days after their admission to the hospital. The tables describing their status on the Brief Psychiatric Rating Scale indicate that as a group they were experiencing moderately severe symptoms of their disorders.

Tables 6.2–6.5 show the performance of the patients compared to the nonpatient group. Most patients performed as well as the nonpatients. Nevertheless, a significant proportion of patients had ratings in

TABLE 6.1. Sample Description for MacCAT-T Study

Variables	Patients Hospitalized With Schizophrenia N = 40	Community (non-ill) N = 40
Age (mean)	39.1	39.0
(S.D.)	9.6	9.9
Male (%)	80	80
White	85	85
Socioeconomic level (IV–V) (%)	87	80
Schizophrenia or schizoaffective disorder (%)	100	0
Involuntary commitment (%)	23	NA
Days from admission to testing (mean)	4.2	NA
Number of prior admissions, 3 or more (%)	85	NA
BPRS total (mean)	50.2	NA
(S.D.)	(8.5)	

BPRS = brief psychiatric rating scale; S.D. = standard deviation.

TABLE 6.2. Frequencies and Percentages for Understanding Scores

Score	Hospital		Community	
	N	%	N	%
Understanding 1 (Disorder)				
2.00–1.70	18	45.0	32	80.0
1.69–1.30	9	22.5	6	15.0
1.29–1.00	7	17.5	2	5.0
< 1.00	6	15.0	0	0.0
Mean		1.46		1.83
S.D.		.60		.23
Understanding 2 (Treatment)				
2.00–1.70	26	65.0	37	92.5
1.69–1.30	9	22.5	2	5.0
1.29–1.00	1	2.5	0	0.0
< 1.00	4	10.0	2	5.0
Mean		1.66		1.94
S.D.		.55		.24
Understanding 3 (Benefits/Risks)				
2.00–1.70	10	25.0	31	77.5
1.69–1.30	7	17.5	5	12.5
1.29–1.00	13	32.5	3	7.5
< 1.00	10	25.0	1	2.5
Mean		1.20		1.83
S.D.		.56		.34
Understanding total				
6.0–5.1	13	32.5	36	90.0
5.0–4.1	14	35.0	2	5.0
4.0–3.1	6	5.0	2	5.0
3.0–2.1	5	12.5	0	0.0
< 2.1	2	5.0	0	0.0
Mean		4.33		5.60
S.D.		1.35		.66

$t = 5.19; p = .000$

TABLE 6.3. Frequencies and Percentages for Appreciation Scores

	Hospital	
Variables	N	%
Appreciation I (Disorder)		
Full credit (2)	31	77.5
Partial credit (1)	4	10.0
No credit (0)	5	12.5
Appreciation 2 (Treatment)		
Full credit (2)	36	90.0
Partial credit (1)	1	2.5
No credit (0)	3	7.5
Appreciation total		
Full credit (4)	31	77.5
(3)	2	5.0
Partial credit (2)	3	7.5
(1)	3	7.5
No credit (0)	1	2.5

the bottom range of the scales, well below the nonpatients. These tables provide a point of comparison with which clinicians can form opinions about the significance of deficits on the MacCAT-T for their own patients. For example, if a clinician's ratings for a patient result in an Understanding Summary Rating of 3, the patient's rating is in the bottom 20 percent of our research sample and has performed more poorly than any of our nonpatients. What significance this may have is discussed Chapter 7 on interpretation.

Table 6.6 shows the relation between patients' MacCAT-T ratings and their clinical characteristics. MacCAT-T ratings were not strongly related to overall severity of symptoms, but they were substantially related to severity of certain *types* of symptoms. For example, Understanding ratings tended to be lower with greater severity of Conceptual Disorganization and Disorientation on the BPRS. These data may be used in conjunction with clinical assessment of patients to offer potential reasons for their poor decision-making abilities on the MacCAT-T.

TABLE 6.4. Frequencies and Percentages for Reasoning Scores

Variables	Hospital N	Hospital %	Community N	Community %
Consequential Thinking				
Full credit (2)	18	45.0	28	70.0
Partial credit (1)	15	37.5	7	17.5
No credit (0)	7	17.5	5	12.5
Mean	1.28		1.58	
S.D.	.75		.71	
Comparative Thinking				
Full credit (2)	16	40.0	17	42.5
Partial credit (1)	4	10.0	4	10.0
No credit (0)	20	50.0	19	42.5
Mean	.90		.95	
S.D.	.96		.96	
Generating Consequences				
Full credit (2)	24	60.0	34	85.0
Partial credit (1)	8	20.0	3	7.5
No Credit (0)	8	20.0	3	7.5
Mean	1.40		1.78	
S.D.	.81		.57	
Logical Reasoning				
Full credit (2)	3	77.5	35	87.5
Partial credit (1)	3	7.5	4	10.0
No Credit (0)	6	15.0	1	2.5
Mean	1.63		1.85	
S.D.	.74		.42	
Reasoning total				
8.0	8	20.0	1	30.0
7.0–6.0	13	32.5	16	40.0
5.0–4.0	11	17.5	10	25.0
3.0–2.0	2	5.0	1	2.5
1.0–0.0	6	15.0	1	2.5
Mean	5.20		6.15	
S.D.	2.42		1.69	

$t = 2.15; p = .038$

TABLE 6.5. Frequencies and Percentages for Expressing Choice

Variables	Hospital		Community	
	N	%	N	%
Full credit (2)	38	95.0	40	100.0
Partial credit (1)	1	2.5	0	0.0
No credit (0)	1	2.5	0	0.0

$t = 1.36; p = .183$

TABLE 6.6. Relations Between MacCAT-T Ratings and Symptom Severity on Brief Psychiatric Rating Scale (BPRS)

BPRS Variables	Understanding	Reasoning	Appreciation	Expressing a Choice
Total	−.07	−.13	−.10	−.20
1 Somatic concern				
2 Anxiety				
3 Withdrawal				
4 Conceptual disorganization	−.51***			−.26*
5 Guilt feelings	.31*			
6 Tension				−.38**
7 Mannerisms	−.31*			−.51***
8 Grandiosity				
9 Depressive mood	.49***			
10 Hostility		−.30*	−.26*	
11 Suspiciousness	.27*			
12 Hallucinations	−.30*		.30*	
13 Motor retardation				
14 Uncooperative	−.34*	−.27*		
15 Unusual thought				
16 Blunted affect			−.27*	
17 Excitement				
18 Disorientation	−.42**			
19 Elevated mood				

Only statistically significant correlations are shown for individual BPRS symptoms.
*$p < .05$; **$p < .01$; ***$p < .001$.

In our field studies, we found that performance on the four types of abilities on the MacCAT-T were modestly correlated (between .60 and .70). This means that there will be a tendency for patients who perform poorly on one of the areas of ability to perform poorly on another. These relationships, however, are not high enough to be predictive. Often one will not be able to judge accurately patients' levels of MacCAT-T Reasoning ability on the basis of their MacCAT-T Understanding ratings. There will be a number of patients who perform fairly well in one area and poorly in another.

SUMMARY

This chapter has provided information, supplementing the MacCAT-T manual in the Appendix, to assist the clinician in administering and rating the MacCAT-T, a structured interview with which patients' decision-making abilities can be assessed in the context of an informed consent process. The method has several advantages. It assures that clinicians will obtain critical information about all four of the abilities that are conceptually related to competence to consent to treatment. Its administration and scoring are sufficiently standardized to allow the clinician to compare patients to our normative field samples, and with experience to develop a sense of patients' individual differences in abilities across cases. Our experience in training clinicians to administer and rate the MacCAT-T suggests that one can become comfortable with the process within a few administrations. We believe the benefits are worth the effort.

As we noted in earlier chapters, a good assessment of patients' decision-making abilities in the context of treatment decisions is an essential part of evaluations for competence to consent to treatment. Yet judgments about competence should not be made simply on the basis of an assessment of those abilities, whether obtained with the MacCAT-T or any other method. One must combine these data with other types of information derived from diagnostic interviews and the patient's background. Using these multiple sources of information, within the context of the specific circumstances of the patient, to arrive at judgments about competence is the focus of Chapter 7.

7

MAKING JUDGMENTS ABOUT PATIENTS' COMPETENCE

Clinicians who follow the procedures outlined in Chapter 5, perhaps aided by a structured instrument like the MacCAT-T described in Chapter 6, will have collected the data necessary to reach conclusions about patients' abilities to make treatment decisions. Those raw data, however, do not in themselves reveal whether patients are competent or incompetent decision makers. This chapter explains how to use the data to reach a judgment about whether patients have adequate capacities to make decisions about their treatment and how to document those conclusions.

THE PROCESS OF REACHING COMPETENCE JUDGMENTS

In Chapter 1, we distinguished between assessments of patients' decision-making capacities and judgments about their competence. Clinicians can assess decision making, identifying and characterizing deficiencies. The judgment about whether those deficiencies are sufficiently serious to warrant depriving patients of the power to make their own decisions — that is, whether patients are competent or incompetent — is usually conceptualized as a legal determination to be made by the courts. Indeed, to this point we have been careful to talk about clinicians' function as "assessing capacities," rather than "determining competence."

This neat distinction, though, becomes a bit blurry in the real world of medical treatment. As we noted in Chapter 1, attending clinicians are inevitably in the position of needing to assess patients' capacities — even if only implicitly — before accepting patients' treatment decisions. If they conclude that patients lack the capacity to make decisions about treatment, they will often turn to family members or others to make choices about patients' care. Typically this occurs without intervention by a court. Many lawyers, ethicists, and clinicians endorse leaving these routine determinations about patients' competence in physicians' hands (President's Commission, 1982). Judicial hearings in such situations would add enormous costs to the medical care system and delay the initiation of medical interventions. In addition, most people seem quite satisfied with how the current process works. The increasing recourse to mechanisms like advance directives (often referred to as "living wills"), in fact, is fueled in part by the desire to keep these determinations out of the courts.

Thus, although physicians lack the authority to declare patients incompetent as a matter of law, they often have the *de facto* power to deprive patients of control over decisions about their care. (Certain extraordinary treatments, such as sterilization, and treatment for psychiatric disorders constitute exceptions to this general rule. See Chapter 8 for a more complete discussion.) Physicians' judgments can be challenged in court, but that happens very rarely. In practice, the decisions made by physicians are functionally equivalent to judges' determinations of competence or incompetence to make medical treatment decisions.

There are substantial gains in keeping these determinations in medical hands, but considerable risks as well. The judgment of whether a person should lose the right to make his or her own treatment decisions is an important one. As a society, we have struggled to define the standards to be applied to these determinations and the weight to be given the conflicting interests involved. To be legitimate, physicians' *de facto* determinations of patients' competence must apply the same standards and attempt to reach the same judgments as would result from judicial proceedings. The task of the evaluating clinician, therefore, can be conceptualized as attempting to mimic the judgment that would be reached by a court in that case.

Sometimes, of course, adjudicating a patient's competence *will* occur in court, either because the situation constitutes one of the exceptions to the implicit rule that allows physicians to make these determinations or because the physician's judgment has been challenged by one of the other parties. Even in those cases, clinicians' knowledge of how the courts make such decisions is important in shaping the scope of their testimony and the opinions that are offered. In fact, most often it will be an initial determination by a clinician that a patient would probably be found incompetent by a court that will trigger a formal judicial hearing.

As we discuss how to reach judgments about patients' competence, therefore, we describe a process generally compatible with the decisions made by most courts. By no means do we intend to suggest that judges as a rule go through each step of the process that we outline here. Indeed, empirical studies of judicial decision making, although rare, suggest that judges' practices vary and do not always follow the accepted contours of the law. But the process we outline is consistent with the normative approaches detailed by appellate courts in many jurisdictions, and with the views of many of the leading experts on decisional competence.

Framing the Questions

There are no test scores, ratings, or hard-and-fast rules to which clinicians can turn for definitive conclusions about patients' competence. As we discussed in Chapter 2, there is not even a single threshold for the level of ability necessary for competence to make treatment decisions that applies across all cases. The extent of the patient's abilities certainly will influence the competence judgment, but Chapter 2 described at least two other relevant considerations: patients' abilities must be considered in relation to the demands placed on them by their own specific decision tasks; and the adequacy of patients' abilities must be viewed in light of the consequences of the various treatment options with which they are faced.

In this inherently indeterminate situation, different ways of phrasing the ultimate question one wishes to answer can have some influence on the clarity of one's thought about the problem. Asking "Is the patient competent or incompetent?" states the options for one's conclusion, but it does not frame the problem well.

We prefer to pose the question this way: *"Does this patient have sufficient ability to make a meaningful decision, given the circumstances with which he or she is faced?"* Making that determination involves an assessment of the patient's abilities and deficits, as well as consideration of the context in which the patient's choices must be made.

Framing the Judgment

The doctrine of informed consent and the legal concept of competence provide a frame of reference for conceptualizing how one answers the question, "Does this patient have sufficient ability in these circumstances?" A helpful analogy is to think of this process as involving a "competence balance scale." This conceptualization does not bring us any closer to an algorithm that would allow us to calculate competence or incompetence precisely, the way we total up our grocery bill. But, at a minimum, it provides a way to describe what we must do to make the judgment.

Our figurative competence balance scale has cups suspended at the ends of each arm, with a fulcrum between them. One cup is labeled "autonomy," the other "protection." It is in this balance that the judgment will be made, as elements for consideration are deposited in each cup. The judgment will be for competence, if the interest in respecting the patient's autonomy finally outweighs the interest in protecting the patient from the potentially harmful consequences of his or her decision-making incapacities. It will be for incompetence, if the interest in protection outweighs autonomy.

This balance scale, however, does not allow these competing interests to begin on an equal footing. Quite purposefully, we set its fulcrum somewhat off center, nearer to the "protection" end of the balance arm. This allows more of the arm's weight to shift to the opposite side. Thus while the cups are still empty, one cup has already dropped into the winning position; the scale is tipped in favor of autonomy.

This imbalanced start represents society's preference for the preservation of individual autonomy whenever possible. Despite having potential data to the contrary, the clinician's process of arriving at the judgment about competence or incompetence begins with a presumption of competence. As the weight of both cups is increased with the deposit of information in them, more will be required to tip the scales in favor of incompetence — with its intrusion on the patient's right to an autonomous choice in the name of protection — than to keep autonomy (and therefore a conclusion of competence) in the winning position.

We next describe the data that are placed in the Autonomy cup and the Protection cup, respectively.

Elements Favoring Autonomy

The elements, or pieces of information, that are placed in the cup representing autonomy are data documenting the extent of *patients' decision-making abilities*. Loading this cup, however, requires some selection and processing of the available data, if our analysis is to take into consideration prevailing legal and ethical concerns.

Which abilities to consider. This book's description of four types of decision-making abilities provides a structure for the clinician's information gathering about patients' capacities. Although our emphasis on these abilities is consistent with existing law and the approach of many ethicists (Chapter 3), application of the four abilities to questions of competence to consent to treatment is not uniform across legal jurisdictions. Understanding and the ability to Express a Choice are almost universally acknowledged as relevant abilities in making judgments about competence. Appreciation, however, is not uniformly named in all states' laws, and Reasoning is identified only in some states and omitted from many theoretical approaches. Moreover, terminology itself can be misleading. A jurisdiction's legal standards sometimes seem in practice to incorporate either Appreciation or Reasoning, or both, under an expanded notion of Understanding.

Although it is appropriate for clinicians to focus on those abilities that are clearly relevant in their jurisdictions, there may be reasons to take into account the potential impact of an ability that is not directly acknowledged in law. Law in this area has evolved in a patchwork fashion, especially when courts and not legislatures have taken the lead. Judicial standards for competence tend to be extremely fact-sensitive, crafted to meet the needs of each case. As long the courts in a given jurisdiction have not explicitly rejected the relevance of one of the four abilities, there is a real possibility that they will embrace the ability when faced with a case that raises the issue directly.

For example, earlier we described cases in which patients' abilities to understand treatment disclosures are completely unimpaired, yet due to fixed psychotic delusions (e.g., that their doctors are only recommending treatment because the doctors are working for malevolent relatives) they do not believe that the information is relevant for their own circumstances. Patients in such situations fail to appreciate the nature of their conditions and therefore the potential consequences of their choices. Viewed from the perspective of the doctrine of informed consent, which is concerned ultimately with preparing a patient to make a meaningful decision, there is no functional difference between a lack of understanding and a lack of appreciation that nullifies what is understood. They are equivalent in their effect; in neither instance is the disclosed information "available" to the patient's decision process.

Some states (Wisconsin is one) have explicitly rejected the appreciation standard as relevant to determinations of competence. Thus, in Wisconsin patients who do not acknowledge that they are ill are nonetheless considered competent to make choices about treatment. Surely, this is an illogical outcome, and one that courts in most states could not be expected to follow. In the absence of a clear rejection of an Appreciation standard, it seems reasonable — unless informed legal counsel suggests otherwise — to allow patients' level of Appreciation to enter into judgments about their competence. Although Reasoning appears less often in standards for competence in statutes and case law, a similar argument could be made for its consideration, especially when patients manifest a substantial degree of impairment in their reasoning abilities.

Which abilities are embraced, or at least not rejected, by applicable law is not something that clinicians should have to discover in the moments before making the judgment about a specific patient's competence. Such matters should be researched in advance and incorporated into one's general clinical knowledge. Consultation with a knowledgeable attorney can be invaluable in this process, especially if existing legal standards are ambiguous. A hospital's legal counsel also can be consulted to determine whether such questions have been resolved as a matter of hospital policy.

Taking partial impairments into account. It is uncommon for a patient to lose all capacities for Understanding, Appreciation, or Reasoning. Most frequently, some amount of ability in each of these areas will remain intact. (The ability to Express a Choice may come closer to an all-or-nothing function.) Thus, as clinicians load the metaphorical cup labeled "autonomy," they need to be sensitive to the degree of impairment that is present and to its implications.

When assessing patients' Understanding, for example, clinicians typically inquire into comprehension of the nature of the disorder, the nature of the proposed treatment, its benefits, its risks, and the alternatives, along with their benefits and risks. However, deficiencies in each of these areas are not necessarily equivalent. As long as patients understand that they are ill, their grasp of the precise pathophysiology of their disorders — and sometimes even the names given to the disorders by their physicians — may be irrelevant to their abilities to make treatment decisions. Understanding the nature of the proposed treatment is usually essential to an informed choice, but the degree of detail required will vary. Ascertaining that a patient comprehends the treatment's benefits is often more critical when a patient is refusing treatment, whereas assessing comprehension of risks may be more important when a patient is accepting it. The weight to be given impairments in understanding the nature of alternative treatments will vary with their accessibility, feasibility, and likely efficacy. Structured assessment instruments like the MacCAT-T offer an easy way for the clinician to tease apart impairments in these various areas, rather than only looking at Understanding as a whole.

Similar considerations apply to Appreciation. Some patients will irrationally deny their illness, yet recognize the potential value of treatment.

> A 53-year-old man with chronic schizophrenia had always been resistant to acknowledging his illness. When his psychologist explained to him that the ideas he had concerning organized crime tapping into his bank account and altering the content of his favorite television shows were in fact false beliefs precipitated by his illness, the patient demurred. He refused to acknowledge that these were unrealistic or delusional beliefs, and again rejected the notion that he suffered from schizophrenia. His agitation, he said, was the natural consequence of his persecution. "If the Mafia were controlling your life, you'd be agitated too." Nonetheless, the patient was willing to accept treatment with neuroleptic medication because he agreed that the "tranquilizers" might reduce his agitation and help him to deal with the real stresses in his life.

In such a case, the patient's failure to appreciate the nature of his condition might be given little weight, because it is having essentially no effect on his treatment decision; that is, were he able to acknowledge his disorder, his decision would almost certainly be the same. If the patient were refusing all treatment because of his perception that he was not ill, however, or if he were requesting treatment for a condition he delusionally believed was present when it was not, greater weight would be given to this factor.

Reasoning abilities, as well, must be scrutinized to understand the implications of any impairment detected. A patient's failure to articulate clear reasons for a choice may be due to an inability to put into words those factors that entered into an implicit reasoning process, rather than any inherent irrationality on the part of the patient. Not all patients perform well on formal tests of rational thinking, such as are employed in many structured instruments, including the MacCAT-T. Although poor performance on these measures may be suggestive of more profound impairments, they do not by themselves indicate that patients are unable to make competent treatment decisions.

In considering the implications of partial impairment of patients' abilities, evaluators must be careful not to ignore the level of functioning ordinarily manifested by the general population. This is because competence has a normative component. That is, since we want to preserve most people's right to make their own decisions most of the time, we limit attributions of incompetence to those patients whose performance falls markedly below that of the vast majority of the population. In our study using the MacCAT-T, for example, 55 percent of our "normal" community manifested *some* degree of difficulty on Understanding, and 70 percent on Reasoning. Although no equation exists that tells us where to draw the line, in our research we have used two standard deviations below the mean of the population as the point below which we have considered patients severely impaired—and even so, courts might still find many people in this group to be legally competent. Put somewhat differently, evaluators must not be unreasonable in their expectations of patients' performance, given how most people would do in that situation.

Considering abilities relative to demands. In Chapter 2 we discussed the maxim that patients' functional abilities must be considered in relation to the demands of the decision-making situation they face. Those demands will differ from case to case, depending on such matters as the level of difficulty of the information the patient must comprehend, the complexity of the choices facing the patient, and the context of the decision—for example, time pressures and other situational demands. Therefore, somehow the data about abilities deposited in the cup labeled "autonomy" must take into account the degree to which the patient's abilities meet the specific demands of his or her own situation.

The task is most easily accomplished when the patient's decision-making abilities have been assessed in the context of the informed consent disclosure. This is a benefit of methods like the MacCAT-T, and of the kind of clinical interview described in Chapter 5. Because the patient's own clinical and treatment circumstances are the focus of the process, the demands of the patient's decision task are "built into" the assessment. The level of ability that is manifested is that of which the patient is capable given the demands of the specific treatment situation. Therefore, the question of ability relative to demand is already answered and ready for entry when one is considering what to place in the cup representing autonomy.

Elements Favoring Protection

The elements, or pieces of information, that are placed in the cup representing protection of the patient from the adverse effects of an incompetent decision are data pertaining to the *potential consequences of the patient's choice.* The balance is tipped in the direction of protection by the excess of negative over positive consequences. As we discussed in Chapter 2, it is consistent with most legal and ethical perspectives that judgments of competence ("Does this patient have sufficient ability?") should consider the degree of potential benefit and potential harm to patients if their decisions are honored. Doing this in a way that can contribute to the final competence judgment may be the most complex part of the process. The following strategy, however, provides some guidance.

Identifying benefits and harms. The first step in this strategy is to identify a treatment option's benefits and harms. By "benefits," we mean any potential consequences of a course of treatment — which may occur in the process of the treatment or as a final outcome — that promote physical or psychological health, well-being, or symptom reduction. Relief from pain, lowered risk of cardiac dysfunction, reduction of psychiatric symptoms, increased self-esteem, and greater mobility are all examples of such benefits.

We use the term "harms" to refer to discomforts, illnesses, psychological dysfunction or distress, physical injury, or death as consequences of a course of treatment. Side effects of medications, infection, the untreated progression of a life-threatening disease, loss of motor function due to brain surgery, and facial disfigurement are examples of harms. In medical and legal discourse, one finds that what we call "harms" often are referred to as "risks." The meaning of the term "risk," however, is really broader, referring not just to the nature of an adverse consequence, but also to its probability. At this point we are simply defining harm itself. We will revisit the concept of "risk" later.

Note that we are defining consequences as benefits or harms solely from the perspective of medical or social convention. In other contexts, what is a benefit or a harm is a matter of personal interpretation. Death may be perceived as a benefit, for example, by some people in some circumstances; indeed, it can be asserted that people should be allowed to consider death a benefit, and to pursue it, if they are competent to make the decision. But for purposes of describing our process of judging competence, medically and socially conventional perspectives on benefits and harms are the appropriate frame of reference, because they tell us something about the seriousness of the patient's choice. This does not mean that patients are precluded from making medically or socially unconventional choices. As it will become clear, they are not.

Translating benefits and harms to "probable gains" and "risks." Having identified a treatment's relevant benefits and harms, the clinician must evaluate their importance. The key to this lies in considering two factors: their *likelihood* and their *magnitude.*

A treatment's benefits, for example, are not expressed merely by considering their great desirability (magnitude), since they may have only a low probability of occurring. Nor is it meaningful to consider only their high likelihood, as some benefits have little impact even when they do occur. Both factors must be taken into consideration. We will refer to the product of a benefit's likelihood and magnitude as a treatment's *probable gains.*

Similarly, harms may vary in their undesirability — whether their occurrence would be catastrophic or merely uncomfortable. But, especially as they are of increasing undesirability, we want to look at their probability of occurring as well; after all, the chances they will occur may only be slight. We follow the ethicists Buchanan and Brock in using magnitude and likelihood to comprise a treatment's *risks*, which they define as "the product of the *magnitude* of the harm that would result . . . and the *probability* that the harm will result . . ." (1989, p. 83).

Notice that this conceptualization of the risk associated with a treatment allows "high" or "low" risks to arise in different ways, consistent with the manner in which we already think about such things in clinical work. For example, death is usually perceived as a high magnitude of harm; yet if its chance of occurring with a particular clinical procedure is extremely slight, perhaps less than 1 percent, ordinarily we do not think of death as a high risk when considering the procedure. On the other hand, death's magnitude of undesirability is so high that even a modest increase in its probability — for example, up to 10 percent or 15 percent — may be enough for us to consider the procedure as being high risk.

In contrast, a harm of only moderate magnitude — for example, wound infection as a consequence of a surgical procedure — will have to rise to a higher likelihood of occurrence than that, before we call the treatment a high risk procedure. And some mildly undesirable harms, such as the side effects of some medications (e.g., dry mouth with many antidepressants) are rarely perceived as significant treatment risks even if they are almost certain to occur.

Weighting a treatment's probable gain-risk status. Having evaluated the probable gains and risks of the treatment that the patient is favoring, the clinician must form an opinion about the status of the treatment that takes both of these features into consideration. This is facilitated by using a few discrete categories to describe the status of treatments. As an illustration, consider the following four categories:

1. High probable gain-low risk
2. Moderate probable gain-moderate risk

3. High probable gain-high risk
4. Low probable gain-high risk

These suggested categories are not meant to imply that one could not employ intermediate categories (e.g., "moderate probable gain-high risk"); but they are not necessary here to demonstrate the process.

If we think of what we are doing as determining the weight to be placed in the cup representing "protection" on the competence balance scale, the foregoing categories have been listed in increasing order of weight. We will load in a much greater weight when the patient is opting for a low probable gain–high risk treatment than if the patient's preference is a high probable gain–low risk treatment.

Balancing Autonomy and Protection

What is the result when autonomy and protection are balanced against each other? In effect, a low probable gain–high risk decision, which adds substantial weight to the cup representing protection, will require a much greater weight of ability in the opposing cup to keep the scale tipped toward autonomy. In contrast, if the patient's preference is for a high probable gain–low risk treatment, a lower degree of ability is acceptable; less weight in the autonomy cup will be required for the patient to be perceived as competent.

In the framework of our analogy of the competence balance scale, this is the answer to the question we framed at the beginning of the process. "Does this patient have sufficient ability to make a meaningful choice, given the circumstances with which he or she is faced?" The answer depends on the balance of (1) the patient's abilities in the face of the decisional demands, weighed against (2) the probable gain-risk status of the patient's treatment choice, (3) when the fulcrum is set to favor autonomy.

One final adjustment, however, may be required. A moment's reflection will suggest that often our concern is not only with the probable gain–risk balance of the patient's choice but also with its status in relation to the patient's other options. Typically clinicians recommend to patients treatments that they believe represent the best probable gain–risk status among the alternative treatments available. Some ethical analyses suggest that greater ability should be required for a finding of competence when patients' choices represent a *rejection* of the "best" options rather than an *acceptance* of them.

For example, imagine that two patients state a preference for treatments that their clinicians believe have a high probable gain–moderate risk ratio. For the first patient, the other non-chosen options all display the same high probable gain–moderate risk status; for the second patient, one of the nonchosen options (the one recommended by the clinician) has a high probable gain–*low* risk status. Both patients have chosen a treatment with the same probable gain–risk characteristics. But it can be argued that the second case increases our interest in and obligation to assure that the patient's decision-making deficits are not responsible for his or her comparatively riskier choice. We may require evidence of greater abilities for the second patient, whose choice rejects a safer option.

In terms of our competence balance scale analogy, this adjustment to the judgment process is best envisioned as being made with the scale's fulcrum. Recall that at the outset, the fulcrum was set off center, allowing the scale to tip in favor of autonomy. When the patient is stating a preference for a treatment that represents a less favorable probable gain–risk ratio than the available options, the fulcrum may be readjusted so that it comes closer to the center position. The advantage for autonomy is not nullified, but it is somewhat decreased.

In many cases, this adjustment will not cause the scale to tip in favor of the interest in protecting the patient, with a consequent judgment of incompetence. A patient with only modest decision-making deficits may still be seen as competent in many circumstances of this type. The right of the patient to choose an unpopular, inadvisable, and unnecessarily "risky" treatment must be respected, as long as the patient's abilities to Understand, Appreciate, and Reason about the situation are not seriously impaired.

REACHING A CONCLUSION

Our figurative analogy helps to clarify what needs to be weighed in reaching a judgment of competence or incompetence. It also provides a structure with which clinicians can describe to others the reasons for their judgments. In the end, however, the process will not tell the clinician mechanically what the judgment should be. There are no standardized, calibrated weights, and there is no actual balance scale that will speak the answer by tipping to one side or the other. Moreover, nothing more about the final decision can be said. As with most important decisions in life, we must simply make a choice, trusting that the process has provided a reasonable foundation for a well-informed conclusion.

Shortly after the acute onset of severe chest pain, a 72-year-old woman with a 45-year history of schizophrenia was admitted to the hospital. About one year previously, early onset of a dementing disorder had been detected. With EKG signs of infarction, her cardiologists recommended immediate catheterization, followed by surgical bypass grafting, if appropriate. The patient was amenable to catheterization, but indicated that she would probably refuse surgery. Concerned about her decisional capacities, and not wanting to take the risks of catheterization unless surgical intervention were possible, the cardiologists requested an assessment of her competence. When evaluated by the psychiatric consult service, the patient had a basic understanding of her illness and the general nature of the proposed interventions, appreciated her condition, and manifested no clear-cut irrationality. But she would not discuss her decisions in any detail and could not offer a rationale for her acceptance of the diagnostic procedure and rejection of subsequent treatment. The consultant concluded that a court would probably find her competent to consent to the catheterization, a procedure with high probable gain and low risk, since her understanding and appreciation appeared to be good, and there was no gross impairment of reasoning. He recommended going ahead with the procedure, and then, if surgery were indicated, reassessing the patient's choice and her capacities. Assuming no change in her status, however, he concluded that there was a good possibility that a court would find the patient incompetent to refuse surgery, since she could offer no rationale for rejecting this high probable gain-moderate risk intervention. This inconsistency in her choices, in the absence of a rational explanation, suggested important limitations in her reasoning capacity.

This case, as the consultant recognized, was a difficult one. The patient's history of both schizophrenia and dementia placed her into a category that warranted close examination of her decisional capacities. But apart from the suggestion that her reasoning abilities may have been impaired, other incapacities were not obvious on examination. Moreover, the psychiatrist was aware of the possibility of his own bias, as a physician, in wanting to find the patient competent to consent to a recommended intervention, but incompetent to refuse one. Consideration of the likely consequences of the patient's choices, however, suggested that this was probably the right outcome in this case. There seemed little question that the patient had adequate capacities to make a decision with a favorable probable gain–risk ratio. And, although it was a closer question, it seemed to him that she might not have the requisite capacities to make a meaningful decision when the ratio was reversed.

Clinicians will find that, as in this example, the degree of confidence they experience in their judgments of competence will vary from case to case. In addition, clinicians sometimes will disagree with each other about a patient's competence. Although the strategies described here are likely to improve the agreement between clinicians in many cases, they will not eliminate disagreements. When the balance of the scales is close, differences in the ways clinicians view cases — and in their own values — are more likely to influence their judgments.

Value differences may have an effect at various points in the assessment and judgment process. They can be minimized at some stages by standardization of procedures. The MacCAT-T's structure for collecting data and the criteria for rating them, for example, somewhat reduce one source of potential differences among clinicians in their final judgments. (See high inter-rater correlations for the MacCAT-T in Appendix tables A.1 and A.2.) Other stages in the judgment process, however, are not so readily standardized. For example, clinicians will vary as to where they set the fulcrum at the beginning of the judgment process, depending on their predispositions toward the often-conflicting imperatives of patient autonomy and patient protection. The processes of assigning values to benefits and harms and arriving at the probable gain–risk status of a treatment are influenced by individual perceptions of their magnitude as well as their probability. Consensus about such matters is sometimes difficult to achieve.

In light of the inevitable uncertainties and the influence of one's own values on judgments of competence, we cannot stress too greatly the importance of consultation with colleagues on those cases in which clinicians have some degree of uncertainty about their conclusions. Indeed, the psychiatrist in the foregoing case example came to the authors for help in resolving the issues. For other clinicians, psychiatrists in consultation–liaison roles within medical settings can be a useful source of assistance in thinking through difficult cases and in performing independent assessments if necessary.

At times, clinicians will be forced to reach conclusions about patients' decision-making competence in the absence of sufficient data for a reliable judgment. In particular, patients who are refusing potentially lifesaving interventions, and about whose competence questions have been raised, may decline to cooperate with formal assessments of their decision-making capacities. These are awkward situations. Treating physicians may feel some urgency in proceeding with treatment and often have definite views on the patient's competence status. Evaluators may feel stymied by the absence of data directly relevant to the patients' decision making. Yet a decision about the patient's competence must be made.

A psychiatric consultant was called to the surgical service in the middle of the night to evaluate the competence of an 87-year-old woman with abdominal pain. The surgeons were afraid that she might have a perforated diverticulum. Two weeks earlier, the patient had been hospitalized for evaluation of a mixed dementia and depression. When the surgeons sought her consent to exploratory laparotomy and repair of the presumed perforation, she refused. On examination, the patient was irritable and not terribly forthcoming. She said she didn't want the surgery, but would not discuss her reasons. She identified the year, but not the day or date, and maintained that she didn't know where she was, although with some coaxing she was able to say that she was in a hospital. The consultant was unable to tell whether the patient was genuinely disoriented or merely irritable and trying to put her off. At this point, the patient refused to say anything more. The psychiatrist felt that she did not have enough information to determine whether the patient was competent.

As we indicated in Chapter 5, it is often possible for a clinician assessing a patient's competence in such circumstances to obtain a great deal of information from third parties. Family members and friends, nurses and other ward staff, and the patient's chart can all often provide important data on the patient's functioning and apparent ability to make decisions in general. Still, a certain degree of inference is required in translating those data into a judgment about the patient's present competence to make a treatment decision. And that inference is not always easy to make.

We suggest a simple decision rule for the evaluator in this situation: do not begin with the usual presumption of a patient's competence. Using our analogy of the balance scale, the fulcrum should be set at the midpoint. Any information suggesting that the patient has impaired decisional capacities relative to the task at hand, especially in light of an unfavorable ratio of risk to probable gain, tips the balance in favor of considering the patient incompetent. Out of fairness to the patient, however, he or she should be told that this is the evaluator's intent, and given the opportunity to provide the information that would disprove a finding of incompetence. No matter how angry the patient may be (perhaps the most common reason for failure to cooperate with an evaluation of competence), this notice regarding the potential loss of decision-making power should be adequate to induce sufficient cooperation to perform an adequate evaluation. If it is not, the assumption that the patient's failure to cooperate is based on an underlying disorder is not an unreasonable one. Patients who decline to cooperate and who wish to challenge the evaluator's conclusions in court are always free to do so.

DOCUMENTING THE COMPETENCE EVALUATION

Having reached a judgment about a patient's competence, the evaluator will need to document that conclusion. Documentation will almost always be required for the patient's medical record; it may in addition be needed in a report to the courts. Adequate documentation plays a critical role in allowing other clinicians to assess the evaluator's judgment, so that they can decide whether to rely on the evaluator's conclusions. It also serves a risk management function; if the patient later challenges the decision reached, a contemporaneous note offers the best defense against charges of negligence or malice. Last, but of no small importance, the process of documenting one's thoughts, especially about a process as complex as judging a patient's decision-making competence, often helps clarify one's thinking.

An appropriate note, whether written by a consultant or the attending physician, should include:

- A notation that the patient was informed about the purpose of the evaluation and a description of the patient's response;
- A brief review of the patient's mental status at the time of the evaluation;
- A description of the information that was conveyed to the patient

about the treatment choice, including the identity of the person who undertook the disclosure;

- Information regarding the patient's performance on the relevant standards for decisional competence (which may vary across jurisdictions);
- A description of the potential consequences of the patient's choice;
- An analysis of the balancing process in which the evaluator weighed the relative importance of the interests in decisional autonomy and protection of the patient; and
- A statement regarding the clinician's opinion concerning the patient's competence.

As long as the relevant data are included, the note need not be lengthy. In many circumstances, these factors can be covered in two to three paragraphs.

We recommend that clinicians word their conclusions regarding the patient's competence with care. Once they are entered into a medical chart, judgments concerning a patient's competence can assume talismanic significance. Treating clinicians, now or in the future, may mistakenly assume that a patient deemed incompetent will never be capable of participating in medical treatment decisions of any sort, under any circumstances. In order to reduce the likelihood of such misinterpretation, it is helpful to note that the conclusion is limited to the situation at hand, when that is the case. If factors responsible for the patient's incompetence can be identified, they should be noted, along with recommendations for treatment. In addition to being of direct benefit to the patient, this information will underscore the dynamic nature of the patient's decision-making capacities.

Finally, we find it helpful as a heuristic device to teach our trainees *not* to write, "In my opinion, Mrs. Smith is incompetent to consent to treatment." This wording suggests that the evaluator is the ultimate arbiter of competence. Rather, we prefer to have the note read, "It is my opinion that a court would find Mr. Jones incompetent to consent to treatment." Such a formulation underscores the clinician's role in applying legal criteria to the competence decision, as well as the ultimate authority of the courts to overturn the clinician's determination.

AFTER THE JUDGMENT

In Chapter 2, one of our maxims emphasized that patients' competence status can change. Whether the judgment has been for competence or incompetence, therefore, clinicians, in their continued interactions with patients, should be attuned to any changes in patients' status. When patients have been judged competent, it is certainly possible for their abilities to deteriorate under new circumstances, such as the adverse cognitive consequences of a progressive disease. Even if their level of ability remains stable, it may not be sufficient to meet the demands of a new, more challenging medical decision.

Similarly, when patients have been judged incompetent, one must remember that the judgment was made at a particular point in time in relation to a specific treatment decision. Monitoring the patient's medical progress across time may indicate that the patient's abilities have increased, and possibly that the patient's competent status should be restored. Alternatively, various minor treatment decisions may still be within the capacities of a patient who was judged incompetent for purposes of consent to a treatment with extraordinary potential consequences.

SUMMARY

Physicians have enormous power to make *de facto* judgments about patients' competence. Physicians might most appropriately conceptualize their role as approximating the decision that would be made by a judge, were the case to be presented to a court. The key question to be answered is "Does this patient have sufficient ability to make a meaningful decision, given the circumstances with which he or she is faced?"

It may be helpful in reaching that judgment to think of a balance scale with "autonomy" at one end and "protection" at the other. Patients' decision-making capacities add greater weight to autonomy; the excess in the ratio of risks to probable gain in their decision adds weight to protection. The scale is set to "cheat" in favor of autonomy, given our reluctance to deprive persons of their decision-making powers unless they manifest substantial impairments and such deprivation is absolutely necessary for their protection. Careful documentation of the competence judgment can ensure thoughtful consideration and provide a basis for later explanations, if needed.

When patients are judged incompetent, they forfeit their autonomy to decide about their medical care, the power to do so being transferred to others who will exercise it on patients' behalf. Often the question of who will decide is determined by law. Nevertheless, the clinician has a number of responsibilities associated with obtaining and implementing "substituted decisions" about the patient's treatment. These matters are the focus of Chapter 8.

8

SUBSTITUTE DECISION MAKING FOR INCOMPETENT PATIENTS

When patients lose the capacity to make treatment decisions, unless they have previously indicated their desires, other people — substitute decision makers — must assume that role. Only in emergencies, when there is no time to seek consent from third parties, will physicians be called on to make choices on behalf of their patients. Depending on the circumstances, the judgment as to what constitutes an appropriate course of medical care for incompetent patients may fall to family members and friends, the courts, or to patients themselves, if they have formulated directives in advance.

In this chapter, we review the rules that determine when each of these categories of decision makers will be selected to provide authorization to treat incompetent patients. Then, we describe the standards that substitute decision makers, whoever they are, must apply to reach their choices. Throughout, the emphasis is on the important role that caregivers can play in facilitating the process.

PATIENTS AS DECISION MAKERS: ADVANCE DIRECTIVES

Medicine in the last half of the twentieth century has acquired an unprecedented capability of sustaining life despite serious illness that, in other times, would have led quickly to patients' demise. Mechanical ventilation, cardiopulmonary resuscitation, dialysis, and artificial means of providing nutrition and fluids have allowed physicians to sustain persons who otherwise would have died. Some patients, however, although they can be sustained for prolonged periods, can never be returned to a sentient existence. These include patients in advanced stages of dementia, persistent vegetative states, and coma. Many people feel that the burdens of treatment in such situations outweigh whatever benefits may inhere in postponing death. For other patients, such as those with progressive conditions like AIDS, some measure of temporary physiologic stability can be purchased only at costs in pain and suffering that they find unreasonable.

In response to widespread concern about these situations, interest has grown in creating ways to permit patients themselves to control the use of life-sustaining technology. Typically, such technology will be applied only after patients have lost their competence to make treatment decisions. As a result, a variety of decision-making mechanisms have been developed and have spread widely throughout the United States. These devices, known generally as advance directives, fall into three categories: decision directives, proxy directives, and combined directives.

Decision Directives

Decision directives are documents that express patients' choice(s) of treatment under specified circumstances. The earliest form of advance directive — the "living will" — was a type of decision directive. Developed in the 1970s, and promoted in various formats by different organizations, living wills generally reflected patients' desires to avoid further medical interventions when death was imminent, or when a return to sentient life was unlikely. The effectiveness of these early decision directives was limited by their uncertain legal status: physicians worried that carrying out patients' desires and permitting them to die might leave the treatment team liable to lawsuits from embittered relatives, or even to criminal charges.

In response to these concerns, magnified in a series of highly publicized legal cases, almost all states have adopted statutes giving formal legal recognition to some form of decision directive. Although these laws often provide a formula that the directives can follow, many state statutes explicitly note that other formats are acceptable as well. Statutes commonly specify the use of decision directives in particular circumstances, such as terminal illness. But court cases in many states have recognized such documents to be of general validity. Clinicians should consult with attorneys expert in health law in their jurisdictions to determine the nature of local law. As a generalization, however, decision directives are widely accepted as valid means for patients to convey their wishes when they are no longer able to speak for themselves (King, 1996).

Decision directives have an obvious limitation in that they ordinarily deal with only a small number of anticipated situations. A directive that rules out operative insertion of a feeding tube in the case of a permanent vegetative state, for example, provides no clear guidance as to the patient's preferences with regard to ventilatory support in the event of potentially reversible respiratory failure. One response has been the development of ever more detailed forms, including versions that ask patients to complete a grid specifying their desires across a wide range of circumstances (Emanuel & Emanuel, 1989). Some people question whether patients can make such detailed decisions in a meaningful fashion. In any event, even the most elaborate form cannot cover all the situations that might arise. Another advance directive mechanism was developed to fill this gap.

Proxy Directives

Rather than asking patients to anticipate the choices they would make under specific circumstances, proxy directives afford them the opportunity to designate the persons they desire to make the decisions for them. The legal device used for this purpose is derived from the durable power of attorney, an instrument that designates another person to act as one's agent after the designator becomes incapacitated. Because of questions about the applicability of existing durable power of attorney statutes to medical decision making, almost all states have now passed discrete "durable power of attorney for health care" statutes.

Typically, these laws authorizing appointment of decision-making proxies specify that the designation will take effect when patients' physicians determine that patients are incompetent to make medical treatment choices. (The prevalence of these statutes has heightened interest in the reliable determination of decision-making capacity.) At that point, the proxies step into the picture. Physicians' obligations to disclose information about the proposed treatment and to obtain an informed consent are now transferred from patients to proxies. If patients are alert enough to be informed of the change in the locus of decision making (e.g., if they are delirious or psychotic, but not comatose), there are usually provisions that require that they receive notice and give them the opportunity to object to physicians' determinations of their incompetence.

The effective use of proxy directives as a mechanism for implementing patients' choices depends on patients having shared their desires in advance with the person designated to make treatment decisions for them. Numerous studies have shown that without such discussions even close family members are unlikely to know about patients' preferences or to make the same decisions patients would have made. Yet it is clear that many people who complete health care proxies fail to have such discussions with the proxies, their physicians, or anyone else. Although patients may still be comforted by knowing who will make the choice for them, when they keep their preferences to themselves, they surrender control over the substance of the decisions.

Combined Directives

Many state laws now allow persons to combine the designation of a proxy decision maker with instructions about their desires in particular situations. Thus, an elderly woman with mild dementia might choose her daughter to decide in her stead but specify that under no circumstances does she want efforts made to sustain her life if she becomes so demented that she no longer recognizes those around her. This approach, which binds proxies in the situations specified, draws on the positive aspects of both decision and proxy directives. For decisions that can be anticipated, patients can determine directly what will be done; with regard to the unforeseeable, patients can at least choose the person to whom they will entrust the decision.

Issues in the Application of Advance Directives

When an advance directive is presented, treating physicians may have a number of legitimate concerns. For patients who have long-standing, cognition-impairing conditions (e.g., dementia), the question may arise as to whether the patient was competent at the time the directive was completed. What it means to be competent to complete an advance directive is itself unclear, but analogies to the law of competence to consent to treatment suggest that patients should understand the nature and purpose of the document, appreciate its implications for their future care, and be able to reason through why they desire to complete the directive. In addition, for decision directives, patients probably need some understanding and appreciation of each decision they have made (e.g., no cardiopulmonary resuscitation), along with the ability to reason about its congruence with their goals.

How are clinicians ever to know whether patients — other than those they have assisted directly to complete advance directives — meet these criteria? In many cases, the clinicians will remain uncertain. But state advance directive legislation almost uniformly provides that patients are to be presumed to have been competent at the time the form was completed. The burden of demonstrating incompetence falls on the shoulders of anyone who would challenge that presumption. Were the law otherwise, physicians might be led to undercut the intent of the statutes — which after all is to encourage patients' choice — for fear that they were acting on an incompetently formulated desire.

Competence issues can also arise when patients attempt to revoke their advance directives. This may occur before or after the directives are activated. For example, a patient may declare in advance of a hospital admission that her decision directive declining CPR is no longer valid, or a patient may disavow appointment of a proxy when that person attempts to make a decision that the patient, perhaps in a psychotic state, dislikes. Revocation by a competent patient must be respected. If the patient is thought to be incompetent, and continues to object to the treatment chosen in accordance with a valid advance directive, a court hearing on the patient's competence may be the only way to resolve the situation.

Patients are not the only ones whose competence may be called into question. Sometimes the abilities of persons who are named as health care proxies to participate in an informed consent process may seem inadequate. In other cases, proxies may be competent but unwilling to abide by the patients' expressed wishes. A proxy may, for example, decline to consent to the initiation of enteral feeding or the termination of respiratory support, although the patient's combined directive expressed those desires. Sometimes, overwhelmed by the choices before them, proxies may simply refuse to make any decision at all. Whether incompetence, malfeasance, or nonfeasance is the issue, caregivers have the same remedy. They can challenge the appointment of the proxy in court, asking a judge to appoint another person to make the decisions. This is, and should be, a rarely used mechanism, but it is important to know that physicians have some recourse when the proxy's behavior is suspect.

> A 35-year-old, moderately retarded man was admitted to a general hospital for workup of mild delirium and a fever of unknown origin. He was disoriented and unable to attend to any discussions of his situation. The local advocacy program for mentally retarded persons, during a drive 6 months earlier, had assisted all its clients in completing proxy directives. This patient's document, which came with an affidavit indicating that the patient had understood the consequences of appointing a health care proxy, named his mother to make medical decisions for him. She, however, appeared herself to be intellectually impaired. As an attempt was made to explain the nature of her son's condition and the workup that would be needed, she became angry and agitated, insisting that he be discharged to her care. Hospital counsel were consulted. They arranged a confer-

ence call connecting the attending physician, the psychiatric consultant, and the district court judge on call for medical emergencies. After hearing their assessment of the mother's capacities, the judge voided the patient's choice of proxy and appointed one of the hospital social workers instead.

Another difficult question that can arise relates to the handling of patients' advance requests that physicians believe are unreasonable. What if the patient requests use of a medication that is not medically indicated for his or her condition, or demands indefinite life support, even with no prospect of recovering any sentient function? Patients have never had the right, even when competent, to insist that physicians employ treatments that are not likely to be helpful to their condition or which physicians think are otherwise contraindicated. The same is true for their advance directives. Continuation of life support, however, may be a different matter. This is an issue on which there is profound disagreement in our society. Some significant number of people desire to be kept alive as long as possible, and we have not yet developed a means for denying those requests. Thus, at this point, physicians may well be obligated to respect requests for continuing life support, regardless of their personal feelings about the issue.

Finally, because advance directive statutes apply to all forms of medical treatment, the question of their use by psychiatric patients invariably arises. As long as patients were competent when directives were completed, there is no reason why their choices should not apply to their general medical care. Psychiatric care *per se* is a more difficult issue. Although the matter has yet to be definitively litigated, it is likely that state laws permitting involuntary hospitalization and treatment of some mentally disordered persons would take precedence over their advance refusal of such care, just as they would were the patient able to make the decision directly. (This may depend in part on whether a substituted judgment standard is used to determine whether or not the patient should be treated; see the discussion in the next section on families as decision makers.) Conversely, advance acceptance of hospitalization or treatment may run afoul of state laws prescribing certain mechanisms for making treatment decisions concerning incompetent psychiatric patients. These uncertainties have restricted the use of advance directives for psychiatric care.

Limitations on the Use of Advance Directives

Advance directives clearly represent a step forward in efforts to extend the underlying premise of the doctrine of informed consent — maximizing patients' decision-making autonomy — to the circumstance of the incompetent patient. Moreover, advance directives vastly simplify the task of the treating physician in determining to whom to turn for a medical decision. But they are not panaceas, and it is important to keep their limitations in mind.

The most important limit on the use of advance directives is the most obvious: patients must complete them before they are needed. A 1990 federal law, the Patient Self-Determination Act, requires all medical facilities and nursing homes receiving federal dollars to inform patients on admission of their rights under state law to complete advance directives. Many organizations have mounted educational campaigns to encourage everyone, but especially the elderly, to designate a proxy or specify the decisions they want to be made on their behalf. Nonetheless, surveys indicate that under 20 percent of hospitalized patients have completed advance directives, and often when they have, the forms are inaccessible at the time of hospitalization. Patients say that they would like their physicians to discuss with them their options concerning advance directives, but most doctors respond that they simply do not have the time to do it.

Moreover, even when patients have taken the time to fill out advance directives, there are ways in which the documents fall short of fully protecting patients' decisional autonomy. To make a meaningful treatment decision inevitably means being situated so as to take into account the multifaceted variables that are part of every medical situation. Competent patients faced with contemporaneous decisions can consider their current functional limitations, the likelihood of improvement in their particular conditions, the availability of new techniques that diminish the risks of intervention, and the social determinants that make it more or less desirable for them to continue to live, among other factors. None of these can be known to a reasonable level of certainty when a patient makes advance choices about treatment, and it is infeasible for a person completing an advance directive to instruct a proxy about all possible situations.

Efforts have been made to struggle against these limitations, such as the development of extremely detailed decision directives discussed earlier, but ultimately they cannot be overcome. Nor is there any assurance, as some commentators have pointed out (e.g., Dresser, 1994), that competent persons can accurately anticipate what it would be like to be incompetent, and how their values concerning life might change at that point. Nonetheless, what advance directives represent is not the ideal but the possible. Whatever their limitations, they provide patients with some measure of control over their futures, and they offer the medical care system a reasonable way of making difficult treatment decisions.

FAMILIES AS DECISION MAKERS

When patients have not completed advance directives, the usual recourse is to ask family members to make decisions on their behalf. Until quite recently, the legal status of the family in these matters was uncertain, although the practice of relying on them was universal. Examining the issue in the early 1980s, the President's Commission for the Study of Ethical Problems in Medicine explicitly endorsed continued reliance on families for this purpose (President's Commission, 1982). Families, after all, know patients best, usually care deeply about patients' well-being and, more than any other party, are likely to devote the required time and effort to the decision-making task. Moreover, when patients designate proxy decision makers, they are almost always members of their families.

Because of the advantages of having families involved in the process, a number of states have recently passed statutes formalizing their status. In other states, the courts have acknowledged the legitimacy of family participation as surrogate decision makers. Some of the new laws also specify which members of the family have priority as decision makers. Typically, spouses are looked to first, then adult children, parents, siblings, and more distant relations. Except in the circumstances outlined later in this section, physicians should not hesitate to rely on family members.

Selecting the Decision Maker

Once it is clear that patients are not competent to make their own decisions, and that no advance directives exist, the family can be approached to assume the decision-making role. If state law fails to specify the order of priority, the first task is to identify the family member who will serve as the decision maker. Sometimes the choice will be clear; for example, when the patient's competent spouse is at the bedside, or when a widowed patient has only one adult child. In other cases, however, there will be several family members with the same degree of kinship (e.g., three brothers), or a less closely related person will appear to be more involved in the patient's care (e.g., a granddaughter visits regularly and is in touch with the treating physicians, whereas the patient's children are not on the scene).

When the choice is not obvious, it is probably best to ask family members for their designee as decision maker. Most families are able to agree on a reasonable choice. They may select, for example, the son who lives closest to the hospital and thus is most likely to be available on an urgent basis. Some families will want to make decisions as a group, which is acceptable, as long as they designate a single member to act as spokesperson and point of contact. When there are a number of concerned family members, it can be helpful to convene a group meeting at which the clinicians are present to explain the patient's status and the choices that have to be made. Simply on a pragmatic basis, this approach minimizes the time spent talking separately to multiple family members and reduces the opportunity for miscommunication as diagnoses, prognoses, and recommendations for treatment are passed around the family.

Issues in Family Decision Making

Most of the time, family decision making goes smoothly. A variety of problems, however, can occur. For example, family members may disagree among themselves on the proper course of treatment. In the absence of a statutory list of decision makers, or when family members of equal status are on opposing sides, dissension of this sort can threaten to bring decisions about medical treatment to a halt. A striking example of this dilemma has been dubbed the "daughter from California syndrome" (Molloy, Clarnette, Braun, Eisemann, & Sneiderman, 1991). The original description involved a daughter who, having rarely seen her mother or previously expressed interest in her care, flew across the country to object to her sister's approval of a Do Not Resuscitate order for the patient. Permutations of all sorts occur; in California, we are told, the phenomenon is called the "daughter from New York syndrome."

The best response to intrafamilial conflict is to bring all parties together for an explanation of the situation (as disagreements are often based on divergent understandings of some aspect of the patient's condition), and an effort at resolving differences. The consultation–liaison psychiatry service can often be helpful here. A relatively new resource are hospital ethics committees, which provide neutral territory where the patient's needs and family's desires can be discussed; family members, especially if they are suspicious of the treatment team, are often reassured by ethics committee involvement. If this is unsuccessful, however, clinicians may have to resort to the courts.

A 92-year-old woman was admitted in congestive heart failure. She requested that a Do Not Resuscitate (DNR) order be written for her, as she had previously been resuscitated and did not want to go through it again. Although competent on admission, her status deteriorated in the hospital. Several days later, her granddaughter, a physician from California (honest!), called to demand that the order be rescinded, as it could not have reflected the patient's competent wishes. After some talk of litigation, the granddaughter requested that the hospital ethics committee be convened. A meeting was scheduled, with the granddaughter patched in by speakerphone. She related her belief that the choice for a DNR order could not have reflected the views of the "real" patient, who had been having so much pleasure from her great-grandchildren. A psychiatrist described his evaluation of the patient as competent when the decision was made. After a good deal of discussion, the committee arrived at a recommendation that the patient's choice be respected. In a subsequent conversation, the physician/granddaughter said that she understood the basis for the committee's conclusion, and indicated that, had she been serving on the committee, she probably would have concurred.

Family members can sometimes also find themselves paralyzed by concern over making the right choice, and thereby be unable to make any choice at all. Given what we know about the intensity and complexity of familial dynamics, it should not be surprising to recognize their influence here. Children who have looked for decades to strong parental figures for advice may now suddenly find themselves asked to make decisions for their parents. Siblings and other relatives may play out old rivalries around the patient's bed, each unwilling to make a choice lest the family later exact a price for having done so. Particularly when decisions involve the termination of life support, it is perfectly understandable why family members may want to avoid the guilt of having "been responsible" for a loved one's death. This may also account for the consistent finding that surrogate decision makers are more aggressive in selecting treatment options that would sustain the life of their loved ones than they are in describing what they would choose for themselves.

Physicians who are sensitive to these issues can be helpful in pointing out the realities of the patient's prognosis and (as is often the case) likely demise. These decisions are often not about whether a loved one will die but whether it makes sense to prolong a nonsentient life for a brief period at the cost of the patient's physical suffering, anguish to the family, and the expenditure of scarce resources. A strong recommendation from the physician regarding the appropriate action—

which is entirely consistent with the family member retaining ultimate decisional authority — usually comes as a great relief, as it allows
the family member to avoid psychological responsibility for the outcome.

THE COURTS AS DECISION MAKERS

Courts are the decision makers of last resort in medical treatment
situations. Because of the time and cost involved in pursuing court
review, this mechanism is invoked only when other means of reaching
a decision about patients' treatment have failed. This is as it should
be. When patients have made their own decisions in advance or selected someone to make choices on their behalf, there is no need for
the courts to become involved. Even in the absence of advance directives, judicial review is not required as long as appropriate family
members can make decisions on patients' behalf. It is unlikely, in the
usual case, that a judge who has never met an incompetent patient
would be better situated to make a decision about that person's care
than a competent, well-intentioned relative who has been involved in
the patient's life. There are, however, circumstances in which judicial
involvement is unavoidable.

Patients With Advance Directives

Completion of an advance directive does not necessarily eliminate the
possibility that the case of an incompetent patient will end up in
court. Patients who are thought to be incompetent because of psychosis, dementia, delirium, or other conditions that do not rob them
of consciousness may disagree with their physicians' judgment of their
capacities. Most states' advance directive statutes allow patients to
challenge in court the determination of their incompetence, and elsewhere patients have this right on a common-law basis. The court's task
in these cases is only to determine competence, usually after hearing
testimony from physicians involved in the patient's care. If a judge
concurs in the physicians' judgment, the advance directive is invoked

and whoever has been named as proxy begins making decisions for the patient. As noted earlier, incompetence or dereliction of duty by the proxy can also be challenged in court, with appointment of a new proxy as the remedy, as can attempts by a presumptively incompetent patient to revoke an advance directive.

Patients Without Advance Directives

Selection of a decision maker for the patient without an advance directive is not always straightforward. Some patients have no known family members, or at least none who are willing to become involved in their care. On occasion, in such cases, hospitals have been willing to accept decisions made by friends or acquaintances, including landlords, social workers, and other people not intimately involved in patients' lives. The legitimacy of these practices is questionable. Even the legal status of nonmarried partners of the same or opposite gender is unclear in most states. Except in emergencies, when consent will be implied, many facilities turn to the courts to adjudicate incompetence and appoint a decision maker.

Even for the courts, finding someone to serve as proxy for a patient without family or friends may not be a simple matter. For people with funds to pay a guardian, appointment of an attorney to fill that role is possible. Courts usually have a list of lawyers willing to accept these assignments. To deal with indigents, a small number of states have established agencies called "public guardians." In states without public guardians, judges may ask attorneys to donate their time, or they may appoint a social worker or other professional from the facility treating the patient but who is not directly involved in the patient's care as decision maker. When the patient's medical needs are urgent, but there is still time for consultation with the court, judges themselves may authorize treatment. In many areas, the local courts will designate a judge to be on call at all times for such cases.

Courts may also become involved when more than one family member seeks to exercise choice on the patient's behalf. These situations often come about when long-standing family tensions are transferred to the question of what treatment is appropriate for an incompetent family member. Statutes indicating which family members have priority in decision making can help to resolve these confrontations, but only a small number of states have such laws. In their absence, or when family members of equal status are in conflict, there may be no recourse other than to the courts. The question of who is best suited to make a decision on behalf of the patient should, in principle, be determined independent of the treatment choices at issue (e.g., whether mechanical ventilation should be continued), but in practice the two questions tend to become intertwined. Physicians and other health professionals are best off not taking sides in these matters, as they will have to work with whomever is selected by the court.

The husband and son of a 76-year-old woman with advanced Alzheimer's disease had long been estranged from each other. The patient was admitted to a hospital for treatment of a hip fracture, and soon developed a secondary complication of pneumonia. As her respiratory status declined, the treatment team was faced with the decision of whether to place her on a respirator. In the absence of an advance directive, her husband asked that artifical ventilation not be used, even if that would lead to her death. He maintained that this was consistent with the patient's wishes as expressed earlier in her illness. When the son arrived on the scene from out of town and learned of the father's request, he became furious with his father and the treatment team, demanding that they do everything possible to sustain his mother's life, something that he claimed his mother would have wanted. The team was uncertain how to proceed, particularly when the son threatened to sue them if his mother died. A decision was made to seek court review. At the hearing, the husband was designated as the patient's guardian with the power to make medical treatment decisions. She died not long thereafter.

Decisions About "Extraordinary" Treatments

As the law of substituted decision making has evolved over the centuries, certain classes of decisions have been reserved to the courts. Even judicially appointed guardians, for example, lack the authority to consent to treatments that are considered beyond the bounds of ordinary medical care. These "extraordinary" treatments, depending on the law of a particular jurisdiction, may include abortion, sterilization, and psychosurgery. Each of these is seen as an irreversible procedure that may be performed for reasons other than the patient's best interests, and thus requires special oversight by the courts. Sterilization of incompetent mentally retarded women is probably the issue that most frequently calls for this sort of judicial review. Participation in research projects, even if they involve the provision of treatment, may be dealt with similarly.

Due to concerns about the effects of some treatments for psychiatric disorders — most notably antipsychotic medications and electroconvulsive therapy — most states deal with these as categories of "extraordinary" treatment. The option of turning to family members for consent if patients are incompetent usually does not exist. Instead, a variety of procedures have been established, ranging from review by a second physician, to involvement of a clinical/administrative review board, to judicial determination of incompetence with appointment of a guardian empowered to make the decision, to a requirement that the court itself decide whether or not treatment should take place. Psychiatric clinicians often object to their treatments being singled out as "extraordinary" and handled differently from the rest of medical care. This is, however, the legacy of decades of neglect of mentally ill persons in state and private facilities, as a consequence of which judges and legislators have decided that special protections are needed.

HOW SHOULD DECISIONS BE MADE?

To this point, we have considered the identity of the decision makers for incompetent patients. Law and ethics, however, have both been equally concerned with the standard to be applied to medical treatment decisions. That is, on what basis should substitute decision makers — regardless of their identity — decide which course of treatment to select? A rough consensus on this issue has evolved over the last decade, although there are states that constitute exceptions to the

REFERENCES

Appelbaum PS, Grisso T: Assessing patients' capacities to consent to treatment. N Engl J Med 319:1635–1638, 1988.

Appelbaum PS, Grisso T: The MacArthur Treatment Competence Study, I: Mental illness and competence to consent to treatment. Law Hum Behav 19:105–126, 1995.

Appelbaum PS, Lidz CW, Meisel A: *Informed Consent: Legal Theory and Clinical Practice.* New York: Oxford University Press, 1987.

Appelbaum PS, Roth LH: Treatment refusals in medical hospitals, in *Making Health Care Decisions, Volume 2,* Appendix. Washington, DC: President's Commission for the Study of Ethical Problems in Medicine and Biomedical and Behavioral Research, 1982.

Bean G, Nishisato S, Rector NA, Glancy G: The psychometric properties of the Competency Interview Schedule. Can J Psychiatry 39:368–376, 1994.

Berg JW, Appelbaum PS, Grisso T: Constructing competence: Formulating standards of legal competence to make medical decisions. Rutgers Law Rev 48:345–396, 1996.

British Law Commission: *Mentally Incapacitated Adults and Decision-Making: Medical Treatment and Research.* London: Author, 1995.

Buchanan AE, Brock DW: *Deciding for Others: The Ethics of Surrogate Decision Making.* Cambridge, England: Cambridge University Press, 1989.

Clare L, McKenna P, Mortimer A, Baddeley A: Memory in schizophrenia: What is impaired and what is preserved? Neuropsychologia 31:1225–1241, 1993.

Cutter MAG, Shelp EE: *Competency: A Study of Informal Competency Determinations in Primary Care*. Dordrecht, The Netherlands: Kluwer Academic Publishers, 1991.

DiMasio A: *Descartes' Error*. New York: G.P. Putnam, 1995.

Dresser R: Missing persons: Legal perceptions of incompetent patients. Rutgers Law Rev 46:609–719, 1994.

Emanuel LL, Emanuel IJ: The medical directive: A new comprehensive advance care directive. JAMA 261:3288–3293, 1989.

Faden RR, Beauchamp TL: *A History and Theory of Informed Consent*. New York: Oxford University Press, 1986.

Freedman M, Stuss DT, Gordon M: Assessment of competency: The role of neurobehavioral deficits. Ann Intern Med 115:203–208, 1991.

Gold J, Harvey P: Cognitive deficits in schizophrenia. Psychiatr Clin N Am 16:295–312, 1993.

Goldfried M, D'Zurilla T: A behavioral-analytic model for assessing competence, in *Current Topics in Clinical and Community Psychology*. New York: Academic Press, 1969.

Grisso T, Appelbaum PS, Hill-Fotouhi C: A clinical tool to assess patients' capacities to make treatment decisions: The MacArthur Competence Assessment Tool-Treatment. Psychiatric Services (in press).

Grisso T, Appelbaum PS: Comparison of standards for assessing patients' capacities to make treatment decisions. Am J Psychiatry 152:1033–1037, 1995a.

Grisso T, Appelbaum PS: The MacArthur Treatment Competence Study, III: Abilities of patients to consent to psychiatric and medical treatments. Law Hum Behav 19:149–174, 1995b.

Grisso T, Appelbaum PS, Mulvey EP, Fletcher K: The MacArthur Treatment Competence Study, II: Measures of abilities related to competence to consent to treatment. Law Hum Behav 19:126–148, 1995.

Gutheil TG, Appelbaum PS: Substituted judgment: Best interests in disguise. Hastings Center Report 13:8–11, 1983.

Hogarth R: *Judgment and Choice*. New York: Wiley, 1987.

Janis I, Mann L: *Decision Making*. New York: Free Press, 1977.

Janofsky JS, McCarthy RJ, Folstein MF: The Hopkins Competency Assessment Test: A brief method for evaluating patients' capacity to give informed consent. Hosp Community Psychiatry 43:132–135, 1992.

King NNP: *Making Sense of Advance Directives*, rev. ed. Washington, DC: Georgetown University Press, 1996.

Marson DC, Ingram KK, Cody HA, Harrell LE: Assessing the competency of patients with Alzheimer's disease under different legal standards: A prototype instrument. Arch Neurol 52:949–954, 1995.

Molloy DW, Clarnette RM, Braun EA, Eisemann MR, Sneiderman B: Decision making in the incompetent elderly: "The daughter from California syndrome." J Am Geriatr Soc 39:396–399, 1991.

Natanson v. Kline, 350 P.2d 1093 (1960).

President's Commission for the Study of Ethical Problems in Medicine and Biomedical and Behavioral Research: Making Health Care Decisions. Vol. 1. Washington, DC: Author, 1982.

Rogers R: *Diagnostic and Structured Interviewing.* Odessa, FL: Psychological Assessment Resources, 1995.

Roth LH, Appelbaum PS, Sallee R, Reynold C, Huber G: The dilemma of denial in the assessment of competency to refuse treatment. Am J Psychiatry 139:910–913, 1982.

Roth LH, Meisel A, Lidz CW: Tests of competency to consent to treatment. Am J Psychiatry 134:279–284, 1977.

Saks ER: Competence to refuse treatment. N Carolina Law Rev 69:945–999, 1991.

Shea S: *Psychiatric Interviewing: The Art of Understanding.* Philadelphia: Saunders, 1988.

Slater v. Baker and Stapleton, 95 Eng Rep 860 (K.B. 1767).

Spivack G, Platt J, Shure M: *The Problem-solving Approach to Adjustment.* San Francisco: Jossey-Bass, 1976.

Sullivan MD, Youngner SJ: Depression, competence, and the right to refuse lifesaving medical treatment. Am J Psychiatry 151:971–978, 1994.

Superintendent of Belchertown State School v. Saikewicz, 370 N.E.2d 417 (Mass., 1977).

Weithorn LA, Campbell SB: The competency of children and adolescents to make informed consent treatment decisions. Child Dev 53:1589–1598, 1982.

APPENDIX

MANUAL FOR THE MacARTHUR COMPETENCE ASSESSMENT TOOL— TREATMENT (MacCAT-T)

The MacCAT-T provides clinicians a semistructured interview format with which to assess and rate patients' abilities related to four standards for competence to consent to treatment:

- **Understanding** of treatment-related information, focusing on categories of information that must be disclosed as required by the law of informed consent.
- **Appreciation** of the significance of the information for the patient's situation, focusing on the nature of the disorder and the possibility that treatment would be beneficial.
- **Reasoning** in the process of deciding on treatment, focusing on the ability to compare alternatives in light of their consequences, including the ability to draw inferences about the impact of the alternatives on the patient's everyday life.
- **Expressing a choice** about treatment.

Assessing these abilities is essential for making judgments about patients' competence to decide to accept or refuse treatments, but it is not all that is needed. For conclusions about patients' clinical or legal competence, MacCAT-T information must be considered along with other information. One must also consider, for example, that which is learned from a thorough clinical diagnostic assessment and mental status examination, as well as the medical and social circumstances in which the patient's decision is to be made.

The MacCAT-T interview was designed to allow clinicians to disclose critical information to patients in preparation for their treatment decision, while at the same time assessing patients' preparedness to use the information in deciding to accept or refuse the treatments that are disclosed. The interview is guided by a MacCAT-T Record Form (Fig. A.1 at end of Appendix) that documents the nature of information disclosed to the patient and serves as a record of the patient's responses to assessment inquiries.

The process involves three steps: *Preparation*, in which the clinician obtains and organizes information (on the MacCAT-T Record Form) about the patient and the treatment options in order to construct the disclosure for the interview; the *Interview* itself; and *Rating* of the patient's performance on interview inquiry questions. Further guidance for interpreting the results of the MacCAT-T procedure are provided in Chapters 6 and 7.

PREPARATION

Prior to meeting with the patient, the clinician prepares the information that will be disclosed to the patient. When the clinician is the patient's doctor, the clinician will already be well informed about the patient's disorder and treatment needs. If the clinician who is performing the assessment is not the treating clinician, the information necessary for preparing the disclosure and assessment process must be obtained from the treating clinician and/or the patient's chart.

1. **Diagnosis of Disorder:** Determine the patient's diagnosis, and write its name in Disclosure space **#1 on p. 1** of the Record Form.
2. **Features of Disorder:** Select three features of the disorder that are most important for the patient to understand in order to make an informed decision about treatments. Write descriptions of these features in Disclosure spaces **2–4 on p. 1** of the Record

Form. "Features" of a disorder that are appropriate to disclose will vary considerably across disorders and circumstances and will depend, in part, on whether the symptoms of the disorder are primarily biological or psychosocial in nature. Possibilities include descriptions of critical biological mechanisms, causes, signs, and symptoms.

3. **Course of Disorder:** Determine the probable course of the disorder if no treatment were to be provided. Write a description of the untreated consequences of the disorder in Disclosure space 5 **on p. 1** of the Record Form.

4. **Recommended Treatment:** Determine the treatment that in the judgment of the treating clinician is in the best medical interest of the patient, and write it in Disclosure space **#1 on p. 2** of the Record Form.

5. **Features of Recommended Treatment:** Select two or three features of the treatment that are important for the patient to understand in order to make an informed decision, and write their descriptions in Disclosure spaces **2–4 on p. 2** of the Record Form. Features of a treatment disclosed at this point should not include benefits or risks. The focus here is on the treatment process — for example, what preparation is required, the medical procedure itself, follow-up procedures, and duration of treatment.

6. **Benefits/Risks of Recommended Treatment:** Determine two of the most important expected *benefits* of the treatment, as well as the best possible estimate of their likelihood. Write the descriptions, including their likelihood, in the Disclosure spaces **1–2 on p. 3** of the Record Form. Then determine the most important expected *risks, discomforts, and/or side effects* of the treatment, as well as the best possible estimate of their likelihood. Write the descriptions, including their likelihood, in Disclosure spaces **3–4 on p. 3** of the Record Form.

7. **Alternative Treatments:** [OPTIONAL] Repeat steps 4–6 for any alternative treatments to be disclosed to the patient, recording the information on the **Alternative Treatments form.** NOTE: This step is not essential for performing an assessment of the

patient's decision-making capacities; the patient's performance related to the treatment chosen in step 4 above may be representative of the patient's functioning in making treatment decisions in general. Step 7 may be useful, however, in cases in which documentation of patients' understanding of all options is desirable — for example, in complex cases that may require judicial (court) review.

INTERVIEW

Procedure

The MacCAT-T interview procedure combines the disclosure of informed consent information with assessment of patients' abilities to comprehend the information and make decisions about their treatment. The interview should proceed in the sequence described as follows. Some flexibility is allowable, however, to meet needs of specific patients, as long as all parts of the interview procedure are completed by the end of the interview.

Style. Throughout the interview, it is important for clinicians to adapt their disclosure and questioning (vocabulary, sentence lengths, pace) to the verbal abilities, level of intelligence, and emotional needs of the patient.

Recording. Patients' responses to inquiries throughout the interview should be recorded in the spaces on the record form marked "Response." Ratings of the patient's understanding, appreciation, reasoning, and choice will be made later on the basis of the clinician's notes in these spaces. The record form also provides brief prompts to the clinician that are related to the more lengthy description of the interview as follows.

Introduction

Describe to the patient the purpose of the present interview, framing it as a consultation and discussion. Indicate that you will describe what you believe is the patient's medical problem and possible courses of treatment, and that you will want to discuss the patient's understanding of the information. Encourage the patient to ask questions as the interview proceeds.

Understanding — Disorder

1. **Disclose:** Using the information prepared in the Disclosure spaces, describe the disorder and its elements. Ask if there are any questions; if there are, answer them.
2. **Inquire:** Tell the patient that you wish to make sure that he/she has understood what you have described. Ask the patient to describe to you his/her understanding of the information — what the disorder is called, what is wrong, what will happen if it is not treated, and so forth. Note responses in the appropriate space on p. 1 of the record form.
3. **Probe:** When patients' descriptions omit information for any of the important elements, use a prompt to make inquiry about what they recall and understand concerning that portion of the disclosure. For example, if the patient does not describe the probable untreated course of the disorder: "Tell me what will happen if we don't treat the problem — if we just let it go." Note responses on the record form.
4. **Redisclose and Reinquire:** For any of the important elements that the patient (a) has not described after Inquire and Probe or (b) has described incorrectly, explain those elements to the patient again, and again inquire concerning the patient's comprehension of the information. Note responses on the record form.
   NOTE: During the inquiry, some patients might respond not by describing the disorder but by describing their beliefs or disbeliefs regarding the information that was disclosed as it pertains to their

own situation. (For example, "Why are you saying I have angina —
I'm sure it's just heartburn.") Patients' *beliefs*, in contrast to their
understanding of what they have been told, are the focus of the next
section of the interview, concerning Appreciation–Disorder.

In such cases, the clinician can move ahead to explore the patient's appreciation, as described in the next interview section.
However, it is very important to return eventually to the Understanding–Disorder discussion, in order to assure that the patient
does comprehend the disclosure, despite perhaps believing that
it is not applicable to his/her own situation.

Appreciation–Disorder

The purpose of this section is to determine (1) whether the patient
acknowledges that he/she has the disorder and its symptoms as disclosed previously, and, if not, (2) the patient's alternative explanations
and reasons for disbelieving that the previous disclosure applies to his/
her own situation. To obtain this information, the clinician may use
whatever approach to questioning is comfortable. The following are
general guidelines:

1. **Inquire:** For example, "Now that is what your doctors (or "we" if
   appropriate) think is the problem in your case. If you have any
   reason to doubt that, I'd like you to tell me so. What do you
   think?" Note responses on p. 2 of the record form.
2. **Probe:** If patients express disagreement with the diagnosis or features of the disorder as applied to themselves, the clinician must
   determine through discussion the basis for the disbelief. The
   basis may be challenged by the clinician, in order to determine
   whether it is easily modified or rigidly held. Note responses on
   the record form.

When exploring the patient's belief, pay particular attention to the
fact that:

- Both acknowledgment and nonacknowledgment of the disorder
  may occur on the basis of illogical, bizarre, or delusional ideas.

- Patients' nonacknowledgment that the description of the disorder applies to themselves may be based on experiences that logically lead to that conclusion (e.g., the patient has received different diagnoses for the same symptoms during past medical consultations).
- Nonacknowledgment may be based on beliefs that are commonly held in certain religious or cultural groups with which the patient is associated, and in that social context the belief may not be illogical, bizarre, or delusional.

Understanding–Treatment

This section proceeds in the same manner as described above for Understanding–Disorder: Disclose, Inquire, and, if necessary, Probe, Redisclose, and Reinquire. Note responses on p. 2 of the Record Form.

Understanding–Benefits/Risks

This section proceeds in the same manner as described above for Understanding–Disorder: Disclose, Inquire, and, if necessary, Probe, Redisclose, and Reinquire. Note responses on p. 3 of the record form.

Appreciation–Treatment

The purpose of this section is to determine (1) whether the patient acknowledges that the proposed treatment *might* be of some benefit and if not, (2) the patient's explanations and reasons for disbelieving that treatment might have some benefit in his/her own situation.

It is *not* the purpose of this procedure to determine whether the patient is accepting the treatment. It also is not of importance whether the patient speaks favorably about it. The purpose is to determine whether the patient is unwilling even to consider (acknowledge the possibility of) the treatment because of confused, delusional, or affective states related to mental disorder.

To obtain this information, the clinician may use whatever approach to questioning is comfortable. However, phrasing of the questions should carefully avoid focusing, at this point, on whether the patient is actually accepting or rejecting the treatment. The following are general guidelines for the questioning:

1. **Inquire:** "In a moment I am going to tell you a bit more about your choices for treatment. But first I want to see how you feel about the one we've just discussed. You might or might not decide that this is the treatment you actually want — we'll talk about that later. But do you think it's possible that this treatment might be of some benefit to you?"

2. **Probe:** Whether the patient believes or does not believe that the treatment could be of some benefit, determine through discussion the basis for the belief. Record the patient's responses on p. 4 of the record form. The basis may be challenged by the clinician, in order to determine whether it is easily modified or rigidly held. For example, "So you feel that it is/isn't possible for that treatment to be of some help for your condition. Can you explain that to me? What makes it seem that the treatment would/wouldn't be of possible benefit for you?"

When exploring the patient's beliefs, pay particular attention to the fact that:

- Both acknowledgment and nonacknowledgment of the potential value of a treatment may occur on the basis of illogical, bizarre, or delusional ideas.
- Nonacknowledgment of the potential value of a treatment may be based on past experience that logically leads to the presumption that the treatment would be of little benefit (e.g., the patient received this treatment in the past with no significant benefit).
- Nonacknowledgment may be based on beliefs that are commonly held in certain religious or cultural groups with which the patient is associated, and in that context may not be illogical, bizarre, or delusional.

Alternative Treatments

As noted earlier, this step is not essential for performing an assessment of the patient's decision capacities; the patient's performance when addressing questions of the recommended treatment on which the disclosure focuses may be used in many instances as representative of the patient's functioning in treatment decision situations in general. This step may be useful, however, in cases in which documentation of patients' understanding of all options is desirable — for example, in complex cases that may require judicial review.

If alternative treatments are described to the patient, repeat the procedures for Understanding–Treatment and Understanding–Benefits/Risks for each alternative. Responses should be recorded in the spaces provided on additional record form pages (see "Alternative Treatments" form, Fig. A-2) in the same manner as with the Recommended Treatment.

First Choice and Reasoning

The Reasoning and Choice portions of the MacCAT-T interview involve a discussion between clinician and patient that explores the patient's treatment choice and how the patient is arriving at this choice. The following sequence of questions is recommended:

1. **Choice:** "Now let's review the choices that you have. First . . . , second . . . , etc. [name each treatment option reviewed earlier in the disclosure, including no-treatment option]. "Which of these seems best for you? Which do you think you are most likely to want?" Record the patient's response in the space marked "Choice" on p. 4 of the record form. If the patient states more than one choice among which he/she is reluctant to choose, write down each of them.
2. **Inquire:** "You think that [state patient's choice] might be best. Tell me what it is that makes that seem better than the others." Record patient's response in the space provided for Reasoning on p. 4 of the record form.

3. **Probe:** Repeat the reasoning back to the patient in your own words. Then engage in at least a brief discussion of the patient's explanation, asking any questions that will help you to understand and describe the patient's reasoning. Note responses as appropriate on the record form.

Consequences

The purpose of this discussion is to determine whether the patient is able to translate medical circumstances of the disorder and treatment (e.g., symptoms, benefits, and risks of treatment) into their practical, everyday consequences (e.g., effect on work or recreation, effect on interpersonal relations). The following process is recommended:

Inquire-1. "I told you about some of the possible benefits and risks or discomforts of [name the patient's preferred treatment]. What are some ways that these might influence your everyday activities at home or at work?" Record response in Consequence-1 on p. 5 of the record form.

Inquire-2. "Now let's consider [name any other treatment or the no-treatment option]. What are some ways that the outcome of that option might influence your everyday activities at home or at work?" Record response in Consequence 2 on p. 5 of record form.

Expressing a Choice

1. **Inquire:** "When we started this discussion, you favored [insert "First Choice" from earlier inquiry, or note that the patient seemed to be having difficulty deciding]. What do you think now that we have discussed everything? Which do you want to do?" Note response in "Choice" space on p. 5 of record form.
2. **Probe:** Consider whether the final choice follows logically from the patient's previous reasoning and generated consequences. If so, no probe is needed. If it does not, discuss the inconsistencies

with the patient and describe the process in the "Logical Consistency" space on p. 5 of the record form.

RATING

Responses on the MacCAT-T record form provide the content for rating patients' responses. Guidelines for the rating process are provided below, as are ways to combine the ratings to arrive at average ratings for various parts of the MacCAT-T (Understanding, Appreciation, Reasoning). Record summary ratings on the last page of the MacCAT-T record form.

UNDERSTANDING

Rating the items. The following guidelines are used to score each item in the three Understanding sections of the MacCAT-T procedure (the Disorder, Treatment, and Benefits/Risks sections).

2 *Rating*

Patient recalls the content of the item and offers a fairly clear version of it. A verbatim repetition of the clinician's description is not required; in fact, paraphrasing in the patient's own words is preferred.

For Benefit/Risk items, the patient must provide a reasonably accurate indication of the likelihood that the benefit/risk will be experienced, if this was described in the disclosure.

1 *Rating*

Patient shows some recollection of the item content but describes it in a way that renders understanding uncertain, even after the clinician has made efforts to obtain clarification from the patient. Examples include responses that could possibly indicate understanding but are too broad or vague to be sure (e.g., for pain of surgery, "It might make me feel uncomfortable"), or responses that contain some specific and correct piece of information but lack some other part of the critical content (e.g., for hallucinations, "I might hear things").

0 Rating

Patient (1) does not recall the content of the item, (2) describes it in a way that is clearly inaccurate, or (3) describes it in a way that seriously distorts its meaning, even after the clinician has made efforts to obtain clarification from the patient.

Constructing summary ratings. For each of the three Understanding sections (Disorder; Treatment; Benefits/Risks):

- Add the ratings for all items in the section.
- Divide that sum by the number of items to find the *Subscale Rating.* This produces Subscale Ratings between 2.0 and 0.0 for Understanding–Disorder, Understanding–Treatment, and Understanding–Benefits/Risks.

When the Subscale Ratings for each of the three Understanding sections have been obtained, add them to produce an overall *Understanding Summary Rating.* This produces an Understanding Rating between 6.0 and 0.0.

APPRECIATION

Somewhat different rating guidelines are necessary for the Appreciation–Disorder and Appreciation–Treatment items.

Appreciation–Disorder

2 Rating

Patient acknowledges that he or she manifests the disclosed disorder, and all or most of the disclosed symptoms.
OR

Patient does *not* agree with the above, but offers reasons that are not delusional and have some reasonable explanation. Some examples of "reasonable" explanations:

- "Another doctor just told me something else."
- "I had all these symptoms last year, and at that time the doctors gave me a different diagnosis."
- "In my culture [referring accurately to the patient's cultural background], this is not considered unusual or a 'sickness.'"

1 Rating

Patient acknowledges manifesting the disorder and some of the disclosed symptoms but not others (those that are not acknowledged being critical for understanding of the disorder or its treatment).

OR

Patient disagrees or is ambivalent about the existence of the disorder or the symptoms but for reasons that are vague or not clearly expressed.

0 Rating

Patient clearly does not agree that he or she has the disclosed disorder, with reasoning based on a delusional premise or some other belief that seriously distorts reality and does not have a reasonable basis in the patient's cultural or religious background.

OR

Patient believes that the symptoms are related to circumstances other than a medical/psychiatric disorder (e.g., psychotic symptoms seen simply as consequences of work-related stress; viral disease as "merely fatigue—working too hard").

OR

Patient clearly disagrees with symptoms or disorder, but with no comprehensible explanation offered.

Appreciation–Treatment

2 *Rating*

Patient acknowledges at least some potential for the treatment to produce some benefit, and the reason given is not based on a delusional premise or a serious distortion of reality.

OR

Patient does not believe that the treatment has the potential to produce some benefit, but offers reasons that are not delusional and have some reasonable explanation. Examples of "reasonable" explanations:

- Explanations that are consistent with the patient's religious beliefs (or cultural background) that medical treatment generally is not of real value.
- Explanations based on past experience with the treatment in question: e.g., having taken psychoactive medication often in the past with little or no benefit, or knowing others who have made this claim.

1 *Rating*

Patient does or does not believe that the treatment has the potential to produce some benefit but the reason is vague or does not allow examiner to determine whether it represents delusional thinking or serious distortion of reality.

OR

Patient is ambivalent concerning whether the treatment has potential to produce some benefit.

0 *Rating*

Patient acknowledges at least some potential for the treatment to produce some benefit, but for reasons that appear to be based on a delusional premise or a serious distortion of reality.

OR

Patient does not believe that the treatment has the potential to produce any benefit, and offers reasons that appear to be delusional or a serious distortion of reality.

NOTE: Failures to acknowledge the potential benefit of treatment may obtain a 0 rating not only if they are based on delusional belief systems, but also if they are strongly influenced by extremes in affective symptoms: e.g., mania, severe depression.

Appreciation summary ratings. Add the ratings from the two Appreciation sections to obtain an *Appreciation Summary Rating*, which will be between 4.0 and 0.0.

REASONING

The following guidelines are used to rate the four Reasoning items (Consequential Reasoning, Comparative Reasoning, Generating Consequences, and Logical Consistency).

Consequential reasoning

2 *Rating*

Patient mentions at least two specific consequences when explaining the choice. The consequences may be related to only one or more than one treatment option. They need not be for treatments or alternatives that were in the disclosure. The consequences must be more specific than ". . . will help me . . ." or ". . . will make me feel better . . ." For example:

- "With medication, the voices I hear will go away."
- "I would be able to walk with less pain."

1 *Rating*

Patient mentions only one specific consequence when explaining the choice.

0 Rating

Patient mentions no specific consequences when explaining the choice, even after being asked whether there were any "more specific reasons why that choice seems best."

Comparative reasoning

2 Rating

Patient offers at least one statement in the form of a comparison of at least two options, with the comparison including a statement of at least one specific difference. For example:

- "With treatment X, I am more likely to be able to walk places than with treatment Y."
- "Treatment X will work faster." (Note that the comparative clause "than treatment Y" can be inferred from the word "faster.")

NOTE: A comparison can be assumed when the patient's reason for choosing one treatment is the *absence* of some negative consequence of another treatment option that is not being stated. For example:

- "The surgery seems best, because then I won't have to be in the hospital a long time."
- "I prefer the medication X, so that I won't have to be so drowsy" [a side effect of an alternative medication].

1 Rating

Patient makes comparison statement, but does not include a statement of a specific consequence. For example, "Treatment X is better than treatment Y," without being able to say specifically how X is better.

0 Rating

Patient makes no comparative statements.

Generating consequences

2 Rating

Patient gives at least two reasonable everyday consequences, including at least one for each of the two inquiry questions. For example:

- "With treatment X, I'll still be able to walk to places I go in my neighborhood."
- "With medication Y, it sounds like I might be drowsy a lot, and that would be dangerous with the kind of job I have."
  NOTE: Everyday consequences must go beyond the consequences that were in the disclosure, and must refer to practical everyday activities or social relationships. For example, if drowsiness is a side effect of a medication, "I would be sleepy" is not sufficient; "I might have trouble awaking and be late for work all the time" is sufficient.

1 Rating

Patient gives one or more reasonable everyday consequences for one of the inquiry questions, but none for the other.

0 Rating

Patient gives no reasonable everyday consequences, even with adequate encouragement.

Logical consistency

2 Rating

Patient's final choice (in Expressing a Choice) follows logically from the patient's own reasoning, as explained by patient's explanations for choice in R-1, R-2, and R-3.

1 Rating

It is not clear whether the choice (in Expressing a Choice) follows logically from the patient's reasoning in R-1, R-2, and R-3.

0 *Rating*
    Patient's final choice clearly does not follow logically from pa-
    tient's previous reasoning.

Reasoning summary ratings. Add the ratings from the four Reasoning
sections to obtain a *Reasoning Summary Rating,* which will be between 8.0 and 0.0.

EXPRESSING A CHOICE

The following guidelines are used to rate the one item for Expressing
a Choice.

2 *Rating*
    Patient states a choice, or patient indicates desire for professional
    or other responsible person (e.g., relatives) to make the choice.

1 *Rating*
    Patient states two or three choices, seems ambivalent.

0 *Rating*
    Patient states no choice.

INTERPRETATION

The MacCAT-T should be used in conjunction with the discussion in
Chapter 7 addressing interpretation of the data. It is important to recognize that **the MacCAT-T does not provide scores that translate
directly into determinations of legal competence or incompetence.**
Patients with MacCAT-T Summary Ratings that are in the "average"
range or better on the norms for all four types of MacCAT-T abilities
are very likely to have sufficient decisional abilities to support a judgment of competence to make most types of treatment decisions. In
contrast, although very low MacCAT-T Summary Ratings will suggest
the possibility of incompetence to make treatment decisions, low rat-

TABLE A.1. Intraclass Correlations (ICC) Among Three Raters, and Person r Correlations Between Pairs of Raters (N = 40: 20 patients and 20 community comparisons), for Summary Scores

MacCAT-T Rating Totals	All Raters (ICC)	Raters		
		1–2	1–3	2–3
Understanding	.99	.97	.99	.97
Appreciation	.87	.72	.59	.81
Reasoning	.91	.83	.77	.75

NOTE: Correlations for Appreciation total is based on ratings of 20 patients.

ings alone rarely will provide an adequate basis for making the final judgment. Considered alone, the MacCAT-T Summary Ratings should be interpreted as indicating no more than the level of performance of the patient on the MacCAT-T interview. As we discussed in Chapter 7, those ratings themselves must then be interpreted clini-

TABLE A.2. Intraclass Correlations (ICC) Among Three Raters, and Pearson r Correlations Between Pairs of Raters (N = 40: 20 patients and 20 community comparisons)

MacCAT-T Rating	All Raters (ICC)	Raters		
		1–2	1–3	2–3
Understanding–Disorder	.98	.95	.98	.96
Understanding–Treatment	.98	.97	.95	.96
Understanding–Benefits/Pisks	.99	.97	.98	.97
Appreciation–Disorder	.91	.86	.70	.80
Appreciation–Treatment	.85	.66	.69	.74
Reasoning–Consequential Thinking	.82	.69	.58	.51
Reasoning–Comparative Thinking	.88	.82	.70	.64
Reasoning–Generating Consequences	.92	.80	.81	.77
Reasoning–Logical Consistency	.88	.77	.73	.66
Expressing a Choice	.97	.89	.89	1.00

NOTE: Correlations for Appreciation–Disorder and Appreciation–Treatment are based on ratings of 20 patients.

cally, in order to describe the meaning of the patient's MacCAT-T performance. This will require the use of clinical observations derived from diagnostic assessment, mental status examination, and psychiatric or psychosocial history, as well as consideration of the decision-making task(s) with which the patient is confronted.

MacCAT-T scores, therefore, are useful when combined with a clinical process for determining *why* the patient manifested deficits in the decision-making abilities assessed with the MacCAT-T: for example, whether the patient's performance represents the best that the patient currently can do, and how or whether the patient's apparent deficits in decision-making abilities on the MacCAT-T are related to (caused by) the patient's mental disorder. In addition, clinical interpretation is necessary in order to address the degree to which — and how — the deficits in MacCAT-T performance and abilities might be remediable.

During 1994, the authors conducted a modest study of the Mac-CAT-T's performance with a group of patients hospitalized at Worcester State Hospital (MA) with schizophrenia or schizoaffective disorders, as well as a matched "normal" comparison group of subjects from the Worcester community who did not meet criteria for schizophrenia. Data from that study were presented in Chapter 6, and data on interrater reliability appear in tables A.1 and A.2.

Figure A.1.

MacCAT-T RECORD FORM

Patient: _____   Clinician: _____

Date: _____   Time: _____   Unit: _____

Understanding-Disorder

Disclose--"Now please explain in your own words what I've said about your condition."
Probe (if necessary)--Re-Disclose and Re-Inquire (if necessary)

Disclosure	Patient Response
#1 Diagnosis	Rating ☐
#2 Feature of Disorder	Rating ☐
#3 Feature of Disorder	Rating ☐
#4 Feature of Disorder	Rating ☐
#5 Course of Disorder	Rating ☐

Understanding-Disorder (Sum) ☐

Other	

(continued)

Figure A.1.—Continued

Appreciation-Disorder

Inquire: "Now that is what we think is the problem in your case. If you have any reason to doubt that, I'd like you to tell me so. What do you think?"

☐ Agrees ☐ Disagrees ☐ Ambivalent

Probe: If patient disagrees or is ambivalent, description of disagreement and patient's explanation.

Explanation	
	Appreciation-Disorder ☐

Understanding-Treatment

Disclose--"Now please explain in your own words what I've said about this treatment."
Probe (if necessary)--Re-Disclose and Re-Inquire (if necessary)

Disclosure	**Patient Response**
#1 Name of Treatment	Rating ☐
#2 Feature of Treatment	Rating ☐
#3 Feature of Treatment	Rating ☐
#4 Feature of Treatment	Rating ☐
	Understanding-Treatment (Sum) ☐
Other	

(continued)

Understanding-Benefits/Risks

Disclose--"Now please explain in your own words what I've said about benefits and risks of this treatment."
Probe (if necessary)--Re-Disclose and Re-Inquire (if necessary)

Disclosure	**Patient Response**

| #1 Benefit | Rating ☐ |

| #2 Benefit | Rating ☐ |

| #3 Risk | Rating ☐ |

| #4 Risk | Rating ☐ |

Understanding-Benefits/Risks (Sum) ☐

| Other | |

(continued)

Figure A.1.— Continued

Appreciation-Treatment

Inquire: "You might or might not decide that this is the treatment you want--we'll talk about it later. But do you think it's possible that this treatment might be of benefit to you?"

☐ Agrees ☐ Disagrees ☐ Ambivalent

Probe: "So you feel that it is/isn't possible for that treatment to be some help for your condition. Can you explain that to me? What makes it seem that the treatment would/wouldn't be of possible benefit to you?"

Appreciation-Treatment ☐

Alternative Treatments

See AT Forms, one for each Alternative Treatment.

First Choice and Reasoning

Choice: "Let's review the choices that you have. First..; second..; etc [name each treatment option reviewed earlier, including no-treatment option]. Which of these seems best for you? Which do you think you are most likely to want?"

Choice _____

Inquire: "You think that [state patient's choice] might be best. Tell me what it is that makes that seem better than the others."

Probe: Discuss explanation to explore reasoning process.

Explanation
Consequential ☐
Comparative ☐

4

(continued)

Figure A.1. — Continued

Generate Consequences

Inquire-1: "I told you about some of the possible benefits and risks or discomforts of [name patient's preferred treatment option]. What are some ways that these might influence your everyday activities at home or at work?"

Consequences -1

Consequences-1 [ ]

Inquire-2: "Now let's consider [name of any other treatment or the no-treatment option]. What are some other ways that the outcomes of that option might influence your everyday activities at home or at work?"

Consequences-2

Consequences-2 [ ]

Generate Consequences (Sum) [ ]

Final Choice

Inquire: "When we started this discussion you favored [insert "First Choice" from earlier inquiry, or that the patient seemed to be having difficulty deciding]. What do you think now that we have discussed everything? Which do you want to do?"

Choice

Express choice [ ]

Logical Consistency of Choice

Examiner's Explanation:

Logical Consistency [ ]

(continued)

Figure A.1. — Continued

MacCAT-T Rating Summary

	Sum of Ratings	÷	Number of Items		Subtotal Rating

Understanding

Disorder _____ ÷ _____ = _____

Treatment _____ ÷ _____ = _____

Benefits/Risks _____ ÷ _____ = _____

Understanding Summary Rating (0-6) ☐

Appreciation

Disorder _____

Treatment _____

Appreciation Summary Rating (0-4) ☐

Reasoning

Consequential _____

Comparative _____

Generate Consequences _____

Logical Consistency _____

Reasoning Summary Rating (0-8) ☐

Expressing A Choice Summary Rating (0-2) ☐

Optional: Summary scores for Understanding of each alternative treatment

Alternative 1:   Alternative 3:

Alternative 2:   Alternative 4:

Figure A.2.

Alternative Treatment (AT) Form

To Record Understanding for an Alternative Treatment
(Side 1: Treatment) (Side 2: Benefits/Risks)

Patient: _____

Understanding-Treatment

Disclose--"Now please explain in your own words what I said about this treatment."
Probe (if necessary)--Re-Disclose and Re-Inquire (if necessary)

Disclosure	**Patient Response**
#1 Name of Treatment	Rating ☐
#2 Features of Treatment	Rating ☐
#3 Features of Treatment	Rating ☐
#4 Features of Treatment	Rating ☐

Understanding-Treatment (Sum) ☐

Other	

(over)

(continued)

Figure A.2.—Continued

Understanding-Benefits/Risks

Disclose--Inquire
Probe (if necessary)--Re-Disclose and Re-Inquire (if necessary)

Disclosure	Patient Response

#1 Benefit

Rating ☐

#2 Benefit

Rating ☐

#3 Risk

Rating ☐

#4 Risk

Rating ☐

Understanding-Benefits/Risks (Sum) ☐

Other

INDEX

Categories from the MacArthur Competence Assessment Tool are capitalized throughout this index.